J A M U

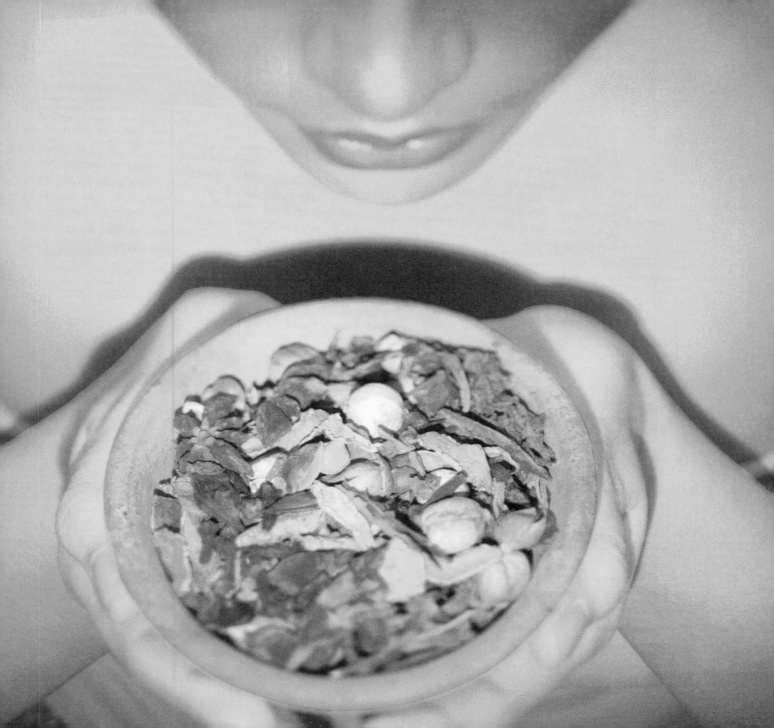

THE ANCIENT INDONESIAN ART OF HERBAL HEALING

JAMU

BY SUSAN-JANE BEERS

PERIPLUS

Published by Periplus Editions (HK) Ltd
Copyright © 2001 Periplus Editions (HK) Ltd
Text © Susan-Jane Beers
Design by Le Bo Ye
Photographs by Artli Ali Hawijono BFA
(pp 2, 6, 56, 68, 84, 89, 90, 94, 96, 106, 112, 116, 126, 135, 140, 147, 155)

Printed in Singapore
ISBN 962-593-503-7

The recipes and techniques outlined in *Jamu: The Ancient Indonesian Art of Herbal Healing* are not meant to replace
diagnosis and treatment by a medical practitioner. Before using any of these recipes, the author and publisher
recommend consulting a physician. All the recipes have been tested and are considered safe, but since some people
have more sensitive skin or digestive systems than others and since the user's actual recipe preparation is beyond
the control of the author or publisher, author and publisher accept no liability with regard to the use of recipes or
techniques contained in this book.

Distributed by:
Asia Pacific
Berkeley Books Pte Ltd, 5 Little Road #08-01, Singapore 536983
tel (65) 280 3320; fax (65) 280 6290

Indonesia
PT Java Books Indonesia, Jl Kelapa Gading Kirana, Blok A14 No 17, Jakarta 14240
tel (62) 21 451 5351; fax (62) 21 453 4987

Japan and Korea
Tuttle Publishing, RK Building, 2nd Floor, 2-13-10 Shimo-Meguro, Meguro-Ku, Tokyo 153
tel (813) 5437 0171; fax (813) 5437 0755

North America, Latin America and Europe
Tuttle Publishing, Distribution Center, Airport Industrial Park, 364 Innovation Drive, North Clarendon, VT 05759
tel (802) 773 8930; fax (802) 773 6993

Contents

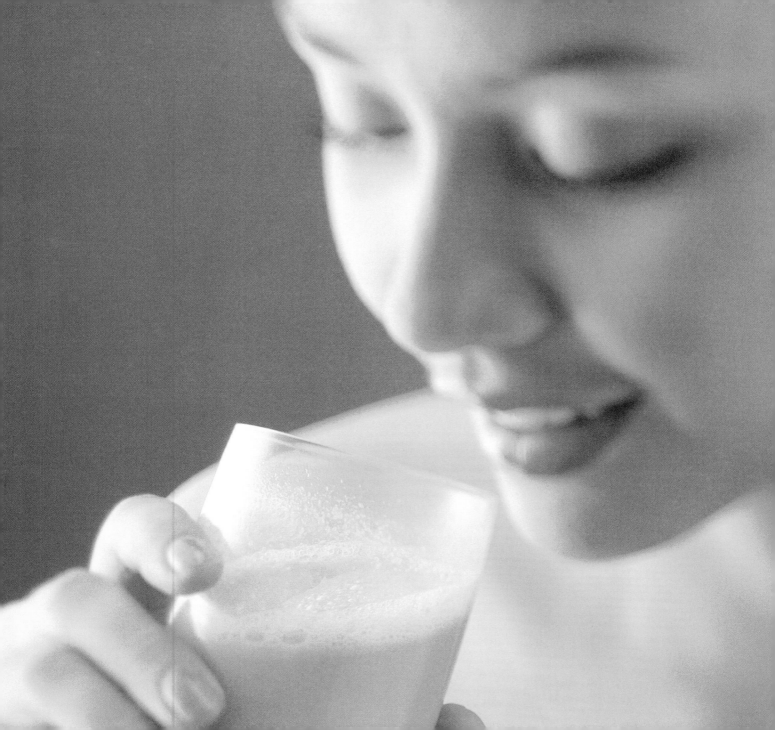

Preface. An Introduction to Jamu

Left:
Drinking jamu every day is how Indonesians ensure they receive the necessary intake of essential vitamins and minerals to keep themselves healthy. It is their equivalent of what is termed primary health care in the West.

Indonesian jamu—part of an integrated system of inner and outer health and beauty, encompassing powders, pills, ointments, lotions, massage and ancient folklore—is unknown to most Westerners. How, when, where, and why were these treatments developed? And, what is so special about them?

To understand jamu, you must know a little about the extraordinary country where it originated. Indonesia's 17,000 islands are home to over 200 million people who speak approximately 600 different languages. The national motto, 'Unity in Diversity', is certainly appropriate in an archipelago where each region still retains its individual customs and character.

In today's world, young Indonesians no longer have the time for old traditions, such as making fabric by hand, playing in a *gamelan* orchestra (a traditional Indonesian orchestral group) or preparing herbal medicines. These were all part of a relaxed, holistic way of life that allowed for any number of variations throughout the archipelago. Now modern Indonesians must come to terms with a fiercely competitive, high-tech environment where survival lies in joining the fast-paced global economy in which we live.

At first glance, it seems that jamu is a casualty of this modern world. Making jamu in the home has certainly declined, but in its place, the herbal medicine and cosmetics industry is expanding and is now producing some exciting ranges of safe, hygienically prepared, health and beauty treatments. The industry was slow in developing, because there was, for many years, a reluctance to share secrets. However, attitudes are changing because rapid industrialization has led, somewhat paradoxically, to an increased demand for traditional medicine.

In former times, mothers handed down the secrets of these healing recipes to their daughters. Those who were skilled at preparing jamu were consulted by their neighbours; and demand eventually resulted in small family businesses. These were the forerunners of cottage industries, which in turn have become today's conglomerates. Now, production has moved away from the home into well-equipped modern factories and it has become relatively easy to buy what Westerners might perceive as mysterious lotions, pills and concoctions in mainstream retail outlets. Also, for the first time, these herbal remedies are available outside Indonesia.

This book gives an all-round introduction to Indonesia's herbal medicines, treatments and cosmetics. All concoctions are simple, practical, exotic and rarely expensive. The ancient Javanese art of health and beauty is a combination of inner and outer beauty with an holistic approach. Although modern medicine and beauty experts seem to have just discovered this idea, the Javanese have practised it for centuries. Herbal preparations and massage continue to thrive because Indonesians know they work.

In the pages of this book you will learn about the closed world of the ancient Javanese kraton (palace) where Indonesian jamu was perfected. You can meet the healers and jamu makers whose skills have been passed from generation to generation and learn about their cures. But if you are looking for a precise, scientific account of inner and outer beauty, you will not find it here, as no such thing exists, for reasons that will become clear. Advice is offered on where to find these age-old remedies, and the Appendix provides formulæ that can be safely made at home. The information here is for people who wish to find out more about Indonesian health and beauty, draw their own conclusions and even try jamu for themselves.

My personal experiences whilst living and researching herbal medicine in Indonesia changed my attitude from one of scepticism to the belief that, if correctly chosen and sensibly used, jamu is effective. This shift in attitude was the result of a chain reaction. Walking round Indonesia's towns and cities means braving heat, humidity, reckless drivers, exhaust fumes and persistent street sellers. These factors, coupled with the virtual lack of pavements, actively discourage any form of normal exercise. As a result of my inactivity, the weighing scales and waistline soon indicated drastic action was required. I opted for aerobics in an air-conditioned gym. However, at the age of 42, my body could not cope with the new regime. Initial stiffness gave way to crippling pain in the knee joints. I then faced three options: stop taking painkillers and exercise with pain; keep on loading my system with drugs; or give up aerobics and become fat. The painkillers won and I kept on exercising.

Then, one day, a visit to the hairdresser changed everything. As my hair was being styled, I noticed a herbal medicine clinic in a corner of the salon. After explaining my problem to the salesgirl, she referred me to the clinic doctor. As it turned out, the doctor was a professor of pharmacy as well as an expert on

Indonesian traditional herbal medicine. My amazement was compounded when the clinic phoned just two days later to say the medicine was ready. I received two small bottles of tiny pills, and was warned not to expect instant results as the medication worked on the principle of 'slow but sure'.

Having dutifully swallowed ten tiny pills for two mornings in succession, I carried on with my daily exercise class, and, astonishingly, by the third day I was out of pain. I simply could not believe it and dismissed this apparent miracle as sheer fluke. It was all the more remarkable as I had decided to err on the side of caution and had only taken one-third of the recommended daily dose. Sceptically, I continued with the same self-prescribed dose and waited for the pain to return. It didn't. Six months later, I was still pain free.

Impressed and by now intrigued, I was keen to learn more about jamu and tried to buy a book on the subject. I could not find one in English, however, and those written in Indonesian seemed to contain only recipes. Wanting to find out more, I took a trip to Central Java where I met jamu maker, Ibu Sri. During my visit she led me into her dark kitchen where she did most of her work. She explained her methods, then said: "You must try my jamu."

Inwardly I hesitated, for the kitchen walls were lined with filthy black woks, or so I thought, until Ibu Sri pulled one off its hook and turned it over to reveal a gleaming interior. Why on earth did she clean only the inside, I wondered, puzzled, until she explained: "Of course we allow layers of charcoal to build up on the outside of pans so they retain heat." I nodded sagely and kept quiet. When my eyes grew accustomed to the gloom, I realized that the whole area, though primitive, was a model of hygiene. Ibu Sri interrupted my musings by offering my companion a tumbler full of khaki-coloured liquid. He downed it in a single gulp, sighed with relish and complimented Ibu Sri on her brew.

Then it was my turn. First I sampled Beras Kencur, which was spicy and delicious. But when Ibu Sri began to stir a green mixture in the wok and scoop ladles of it into a glass, I became anxious. I knew for sure things were bad when a miniature glass of sweet liquid was set down alongside it. (A sugared drink is the antidote served when the jamu is particularly bitter.)

"The Pegal Linu," Ibu Sri announced with aplomb, oblivious to my distress ('pegal' means stiff; 'linu' is rheumatic; therefore 'pegal linu' translates as 'stiffness caused by rheumatism' and is prescribed to alleviate aches and pains.)

Taking a deep breath, I consumed the potion, which made the worst Western cough mixture seem like nectar. The sugared water alleviated the aftertaste only marginally.

By midnight, however, I still had not experienced the anticipated backlash. At 5 am the next morning, I awoke expecting to feel like death, but—to my astonishment—I had never felt better. This was extraordinary—I had actually acquired a new energy; in fact I had never felt more alive and jamu had been the only variation from my normal diet.

From that moment, I was hooked. I began researching the subject in earnest, in the hope that others would benefit from my experience and discover what—if anything—this ancient Indonesian health system could do for them. The result, many years later, is this book.

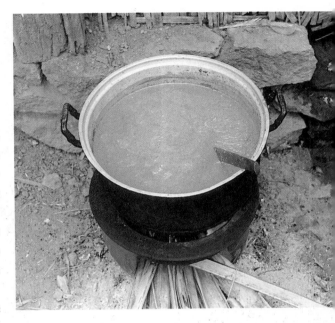

Above:
Central Javanese Ibu Sri was the first person whose home-made jamu the author tested. Here a pot of Kunir Asem is being prepared in her back yard.

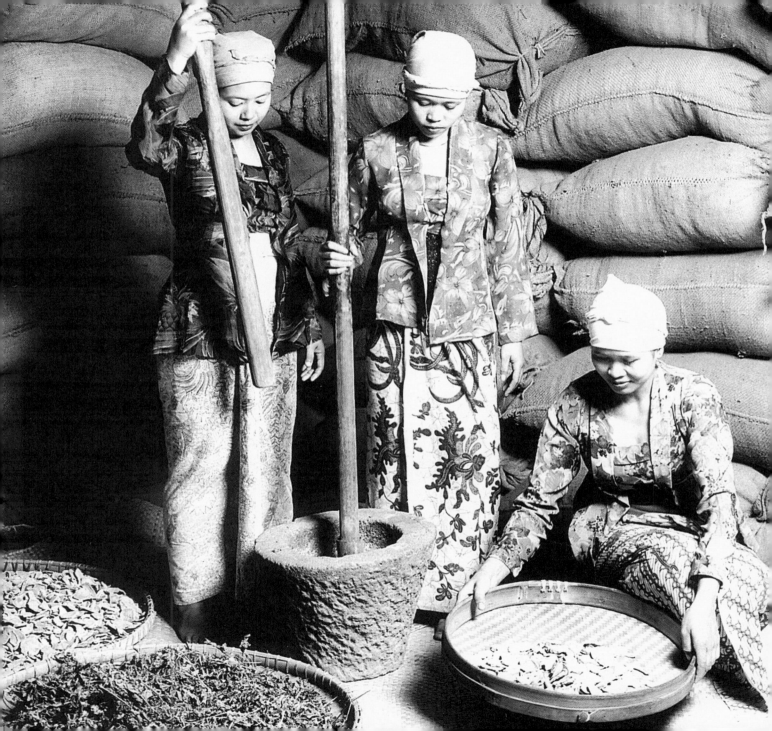

Chapter 1. Indonesian Healing through the Ages

The use of herbs in a curative or health-giving capacity is as old as Javanese civilization itself.

Tracking down the origins of jamu is no easy task. The use of herbs in a curative or health-giving capacity is as old as Javanese civilization itself. Indonesians believe herbal medicine originated in the ancient palaces of Surakarta (Solo) and Yogyakarta in Central Java. The culture of the courts also developed as a result of various exotic influences—Chinese, Indian and Arab—and these influences are reflected in their herbal medicine. But as with many things Indonesian, solid evidence is hard to find.

Early Evidence
Experts agree the use of plants for medicinal purposes in Indonesia dates from prehistoric times. The theory is substantiated by the impressive collection of Neolithic stone implements in Jakarta's National Museum that were almost certainly used for daily healthcare. Tools such as mortars or rubbing stones were used to grind plants and obtain powders and plant extracts.

Further proof can be found in stone reliefs depicting the human life cycle at the famous Borobudur temple dating from c. AD 800–900. In these carvings the *kalpataruh* leaf (from the 'mythological tree that never dies') and other ingredients are being pounded to make mixtures for women's health and beauty

Left:
Archival photograph showing Javanese from the kraton *making jamu.*

13

Advice from Serat Centhini

Still considered one of the major references on jamu, the 300-year-old *Serat Centhini* has plenty of illustrative tales which not only make interesting reading but are also instructive.

For example, it tells how a certain Mas Cebolang went to visit Ki Bawaraga, leader of a Javanese *gamelan* orchestra (photo below depicts a contemporary *gamelan* player). It was around midnight when he encountered an acquaintance called Amadtenggara, who had a toothache; Mas Cebolang gave him some medicine for it. He recommended chewing *kenanga* flowers (*Canangium odoratum*; ylang-ylang) mixed with salt. The story goes that the swollen gum was pierced with a fish bone and the patient was healed immediately. Apparently it was also necessary to choose an auspicious date and time for this operation, to ensure its total success.

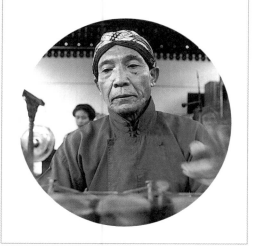

care. These reliefs also depict people giving body massage, a healing process recorded in many parts of the world, particularly in China, Japan and India. With the establishment of early trade routes between Asia and Asia Minor, healing techniques would have quite easily passed from East to West, and vice versa.

At the end of the first millennium, the influence of Javanese culture began to spread to the neighbouring island of Bali, whose peoples had already absorbed influences from as far away as India. The powerful Majapahit kingdom thrived in East Java, controlling much of the seas between India and China; links were established between Java and Bali (a channel of less than five km [three miles] separates the two islands). But the Majapahit kingdom wanted more, and in 1343 an army under Gajah Mada was sent by ruler Hayam Wuruk to subjugate the Balinese. His success was short-lived and the Balinese retaliated on several occasions, trying to impose their rule on the territories at the easternmost end of Java.

Following the adoption of Islam and subsequent breakup of the Majapahit empire in the late 15th century, many Javanese fled to Bali, taking their books, culture and customs with them. There they remained isolated until 1908, when the Dutch subjugated the island. This accident of history means that Balinese healing frequently mirrors that of Java 400 years ago, and here, Javanese healing traditions have remained largely intact.

Written Records

Gaining access to surviving records is very difficult: many are in the hands of healers or their families who are reluctant to let anyone see them, let alone scan their contents. Indeed when, in the course of researching this book, it came to the manuscripts at Yogyakarta Palace, the librarian was not at liberty to show them to anybody unless that person had received permission from a higher authority. Because of their religious content, palm manuscripts are considered sacred and are only handed down to a chosen few. (Balinese healing knowledge was inscribed on *lontar* leaves, dried fronds of a type of palm.) In Java, important information was also recorded on paper manuscripts, but surviving examples are in bad condition: inks have faded; pages are torn, missing or covered in dust; and whole sections have been attacked by mould or insects which have transformed them into delicate but unreadable pieces of lace.

Dating the written material is also complex. In the absence of modern printing presses, hand-copying texts was the only way to make them available to a wider audience and dates were included at the whim of the scribe. The paper used can sometimes gives a rough guide, but identifiable watermarks are rare. In the case of *Usada* (*Book of Healing*), a collection of texts dealing with healing practices, scholars are still unable to determine a precise date with any certainty. There are, however, two manuscripts in the Surakarta Palace library that have been dated, and are arguably the best references on jamu and traditional medicine in existence—namely, *Serat Kawruh bab Jampi-jampi* (*A Treatise on All Manner of Cures*) and *Serat Centhini* (*Book of Centhini*).

The former probably gives us the most systematic account of jamu. It comprises a total of 1,734 formulæ made from natural ingredients, together with information on their use. A further 244 entries are in the form of prayers or symbolic figures

Above:
An example of some of the handwritten records in the Museum in Yogyakarta.

15

A Multi-cultural Exchange

Dutch influence is evident in colonial-era architecture, furniture, some food and even some words in the national language, Bahasa Indonesia. The cultural exchange was a two-way affair, judging by the number of books and papers on Indonesia that found their way to libraries and publishers in Europe.

In the early 1900s, Mrs Jans Kloppenburg-Versteegh, a Dutch woman living in Semarang at the turn of that century, wrote *De Platen-Atlas* (The Pictorial Atlas) and *Indische Planten en haar Geneeskracht* (Indigenous Plants and their Healing Powers), having collected and tested hundreds of herbal medicine recipes before putting them into print.

Born in 1862 at Soekamangli, a large coffee plantation in the district of Weliri, the young girl was educated at a boarding school in Batavia (Jakarta), until the family fortunes declined and she had to return home to help her mother. Jans' mother, Albertina van Spreeuwenburg, looked after the health of all the people living in and around the plantation; as the local people said: "The *nonja besar* (lady) knew everything about medicinal herbs."

In his memoirs, Fred Kloppenburg, Albertina's grandson, writes of his grandmother: "Outside the cultivated gardens ... everything grew wild, but grandma seemed to recognize everything. During these walks, grandma would often talk with the Javanese village elders. She would ask them how the population was doing, were there any health problems, what were they doing about it. Often she would give advice to these people, showing them what herbs (weeds to us) were beneficial and how to prepare the medication."

It was in this environment, at her mother's side, that the young Jans became familiar with the local plants and their healing powers; even after her own marriage to Herman Kloppenburg in 1883, she pursued her interest in herbs. She became the president of a local healthcare society in Semarang, and received patients, and, when necessary, visited them at home. Her name and her reputation as a healer spread rapidly, so it was perhaps not surprising that she decided to publish her findings.

The Pictorial Atlas, as its name suggests, pictorially and textually describes the principal common plants that Mrs Kloppenburg used in her recipes. *Indigenous Plants and their Healing Powers* taught people how to prepare the herbs, and make the remedies. It was first published by Masman and Stroink in 1907, and was reprinted for several decades, with the last edition appearing in the late 1980s in Bahasa Indonesia.

Photo courtesy of Vilan van de Loo
(Kloppenburg Collection, Leiden)

used as powerful amulets or talismans to cure specific health problems, or to protect the owners from any black magic aimed in their direction.

The earlier *Serat Centhini*, an 18th-century manuscript produced on the orders of a son of Kanjeng Susuhunan Pakubuwono IV, ruler of the central Javanese kingdom of Surakarta from 1788 to 1820, is a celebration of life. Three men were charged with collecting as much information as possible on the spiritual, material, scientific and religious knowledge of Javanese culture. The result was a work of 12 volumes consisting of 725 cantos. It is believed that *Serat Centhini* was compiled as a deliberate act of defiance by the Sunan's son against his father, who was extremely devout and who considered anything other than religious works unacceptable. According to the Javanese scholar Tim Behrend, the explicit nature of some of the material may have been calculated to enrage and offend the old man.

Serat Centhini was copied and revised so often no one knows which edition is the original. Some versions are dated 1742 in the Javanese calendar, which equates with 1814 in a Western calendar, but experts say much of the material dates from centuries earlier. Although the work covered every imaginable subject, much of *Serat Centhini* is concerned with sexual problems and includes copious advice on a variety of ailments as well as a number of remedies. Much of its style is fairly earthy and at times it resembles a series of fairy tales.

Yet, despite its basic approach, *Serat Centhini* gives one of the best accounts of medical treatment in ancient Java. In nearly every instance, the remedies are taken from nature and many are easy to administer. Spots on the skin could be cleared up

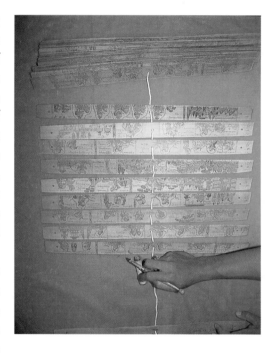

Above:
The Balinese Cultural Document Office in Denpasar has many examples of lontar *manuscripts inscribed with secret healing recipes.*

with a preparation of what was termed *pucung* paste which was made from the fruit of the *kluwak* tree (*Pangium edule*) mixed with *urip* (*Euphorbia tirucalli*; milk bush or finger tree) and *widuri* (*Calotropis gigantea*; *mudar* plant) which had to be boiled up with the fruit. It was applied to spots while warm and was not to be removed for at least one day. The instructions suggest finishing the cure by grinding *elung ubi jalar* (the young leaves of sweet potato or *Ipomoea batatas*) with powdered lime and rubbing this mixture onto the affected area.

In addition to the recipes and formulae, *Serat Centhini* includes a great many stories and folk tales that illustrate the use of jamu in daily life. One such tale relates to a newly married couple. The husband, who presented himself to his bride on their wedding night, was told that his sexual equipment was not up to the mark and that something must be done to rectify the matter. Feeling thoroughly dejected, the young bridegroom set off in search of an answer. He roamed far and wide until he came upon a magic mushroom one day. It appeared this mushroom did the trick, because his wife, as the story went, was overjoyed to find her husband suddenly so well-endowed.

Similar advice is found in other manuscripts or *primbon* in the Palace library at Solo. These manuscripts span many subjects and comprise some 5,000 texts written on 700,000 pieces of paper, which are bound into over 2,100 volumes, some dating from as far back as the 1720s. They include historical documents, political correspondence and court diaries, prophecies, poetry, moral tracts, erotic lore, Islamic theology and law, Sufi lyrics, scripts for shadow puppet plays, court customs and manuals of magical and divinatory practices, not to mention the four sections devoted to 'pharmacy, prescriptions and recipes'. The latter provide detailed guidance on the curing of specific ailments. Other manuscripts contain a prince's advice on sexuality and marriage to one of his children on the night before his wedding. Jamu inevitably plays an important part in these discussions. Indeed, as part of their marriage trousseau, brides were kitted out with a magnificently decorated, square- or pyramid-shaped box comprising stacks of small drawers full of medicinal herbs.

It would be wrong to assume these old manuscripts were only known to the rich and well educated. The contents were usually written in verse and were sung or intoned as part of regular public performances. Those who lacked formal education became attentive listeners as they heard the pieces often, thereby absorbing the endless flow of cultural information the verses contained. In this way, Javanese philosophy and knowledge were spread to all levels of society.

As well as the more disciplined approach to herbal medicine promoted by the various *kraton*, many other healing traditions exist in other parts of the archipelago. A wide range of healing practices can be found in Bali, Sumatra, Kalimantan and Madura, which are also renowned for the use of magic and aphrodisiacs. Java, however, is in a class of it own, due to the all-embracing nature of the cures, their success, and their links to the palaces; jamu from the areas around a *kraton* was, and still is, considered to be the best in terms of status, prestige and—ultimately—efficacy. In much the same way that today's designer goods carry a mark of quality and are deemed superior to mass-produced goods, so it was with jamu.

Below:
A relief at Borobudur depicts someone taking jamu from a bowl.

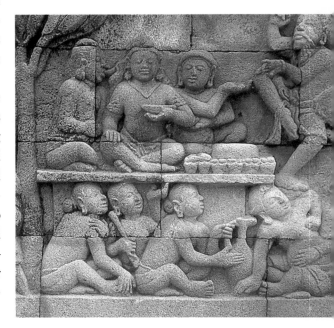

Looking Back to the Colonial Days

In 1968, *Tong Tong* magazine printed an article by a Dutch woman who was brought up in Indonesia. The extract below is reprinted by kind permission of *Tong Tong* in the Hague.

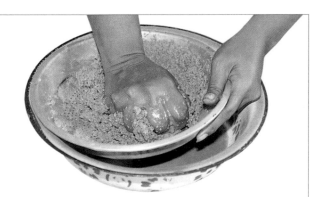

"The article in *Tong Tong No. 13* from the *Indische* (Indonesian Newspaper) of 1910 reminded me of the traditional recipes my mother made from leaves, barks, seeds and roots. When I was a small child the doctor never came to our house because we couldn't expect him to come out for every little illness.

"That's why my mother made her own medicines. She made a compress of *daon inggoe* (devil's dirt leaves) and vinegar for treating severe fever. For sprains the proven remedy was Beras Kencur and for mumps she used a *pilis* (compress) of maize and garlic. She had various cough syrup recipes and if one didn't cure it then my mother tried another. I still remember many healed us completely.

"We usually walked barefoot and often came home with badly blistered and scratched feet. In such instances a *sirih* (betel) leaf was mixed with some coconut oil, flattened to a pancake shape and applied to the sore spot. The foot was bandaged and when this was removed a few days later, the cuts never festered. Some years later, our dentist made an oral rinse using extract of *sirih* leaves. The same decoction was used for ulcerating cuts instead of a soda bath. The result was amazing.

"However, my mother was not a gentle healer. If we were cut by splintered glass, a nail or a sharp piece of bamboo she took the bottle of vinegar and said, 'Close your eyes.' We closed our eyes but instantly opened our mouths to shout when she poured it onto the open wounds! When the bleeding stopped she would put *sirih* leaves on the cuts.

"She also had a splendid recipe for dysentery—a mixture of *kaki-kuda* leaves (small leaves of horsehoof grass or Indian pennywort) and roots of *jambu biji* (guava) with a few other bits and pieces. During an outbreak of amoebic dysentery she made this reliable jamu for friends. A good friend, a Danish doctor, always opened his 'clever' medical book when in doubt. Here he learned butterburr had an important basic ingredient called yatren which was used in a prescription he gave his patients. After that he always accepted a small glass of Mama's curd. Mind you I don't believe that *kaki-kuda* of Begagan is from the Pelargonium family though the shape of its leaf is similar.

"Personally I feel I have received more benefit from the Indonesian remedies than doctor's prescriptions. Once I had an unexpected guest in my stomach—a tapeworm. The doctor gave me medicine on three separate occasions but the worm refused to leave. Then I thought of Mrs Kloppenburg's book (see page 16). I read her recipe and peeled 500 kernels of the delicious *gurih* fruit (*Hydrocotyle asiatica*). First time around I had to eat 200 before food and then 300. I felt awful and dizzy but my guest felt worse and the Kloppenburg remedy won. Quinine was always used to treat malaria of course, but Mama said 'Oh no, *pule-bast* (bark of *Alstonia scholaris*) is better or *meniran* (*Phyllanthus niruri*) and *sambiloto* (*Andrographis paniculata*).' She always had something to help if someone was sick no matter if the malaria made them hot or cold. At that time there was still much malaria and people who caught it shivered so badly they often thought they would die and tried to get rid of it by staying in the sun but Mama's medicines were usually best."

Developments in the 20th Century

Indonesia's medical profession only realized the true value of its natural apothecary in around 1940. In June of that year, a meeting took place in Surakarta that was to revolutionize the future of traditional medicine: the Second Congress of the Indonesian Physicians Association. To coincide with this event, the Mothers' Association of Yogyakarta decided to mount a special Expo entitled 'Traditional Indonesian Remedies'. It is uncertain who influenced whom, but before the Congress ended, a motion was passed recommending an in-depth study of traditional medicine and its applications. This was the first step towards improving the status of jamu and transforming it to complementary medicine status.

The next important development took place between 1942 to 1944, during the Japanese Occupation. The Dai Nippon Government supported herbal medicine by setting up the Indonesian Traditional Medicines Committee in June 1944, under the guidance of Professor Dr Sato, Chief of the Government Department of Health. The committee then appointed the head of the Indonesian Physicians' Association to coordinate with the traditional medicine producers.

Traditional medicine received a further boost during Indonesia's War of Independence. Orthodox medicine was in short supply, so doctors turned to herbal remedies to treat patients. Later, Indonesia's newly installed President Sukarno issued the Proclamation of Independence, which stated that the nation must be self-supporting. In accordance with this directive, imported, modern drugs became extremely difficult to obtain and people were thrown back on their own resources.

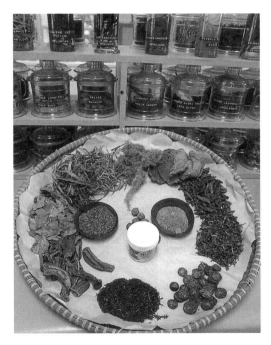

Above:
Raw ingredients and formulae in a jamu manufacturer's laboratory in Jakarta.

Many returned to their parents' and grandparents' age-old, tried-and-tested remedies. Since that time, interest in traditional medicine has blossomed, and a whole series of conferences, exhibitions, seminars and scientific studies have been organized.

During the last two decades of the 20th century, development of Indonesia's traditional medicine industry accelerated. Frequently under siege from politics, competition from imported drugs and a severe shortage of funding for research, the industry has always returned in force following each setback. To introduce some order to the unregulated industry, steps have been taken to implement modern, clinical trials to back performance claims with scientific data, and to standardize the burgeoning industry in such a way that it may be accepted nationally and considered on an international level. With the creation of eight herbal medicine testing centres in the early 1980s, the endorsement of further research centres and the growing interest amongst medical professionals, the foundations are now in place for international recognition of jamu.

This process has been further helped by an increased demand for jamu from outside Indonesia's borders, especially in the developed world, which in turn reflects a general trend towards more natural methods of preventative medicine. Alternative therapies are no longer treated with the suspicion they received even a decade ago; in fact, therapies such as acupuncture, Reiki, acupressure, massage, the taking of herbal teas and elixirs, have become—if not mainstream—certainly perfectly acceptable. All this is good news for those who want to see Indonesia's herbal medicine out in the open—and available in the wider world.

An Interview with Soedarmilah Soeparto of Jamu Darmi

Soedarmilah Soeparto is the name behind Jamu Darmi (see story on page 155), a small but successful and well respected jamu production company located in a suburb of Central Jakarta. As with many such companies, it grows its own supply of medicinal herbs (see below right). In a question and answer session taken from her lectures, the founder answered some commonly-asked questions about jamu.

Does jamu have any harmful side effects?
There are no side effects or harm because genuine jamu is made only of herbs, unadulterated by chemicals and artificial fillings, not spoiled by modern processing. The natural balance of the active enzymes and vitamins gives the human body its wholesome effect.

Is it all right to take different types of jamu?
Depending on your needs, it is perfectly all right to combine jamu intake. For example, a woman who intends to lose weight can alternate between Galian Lansing and Kempes Perut.

Is it dangerous to go above the recommended dose?
No. The recommended dosage is usually the minimum dosage that will allow the jamu to take effect quickly. For quicker results, a higher dose can be taken without harm. However, in cases like Kempes Perut, very high doses can cause diarrhoea. A reduction in the dose is required if the jamu causes diarrhoea.

Is jamu heaty?
Complaints about heatiness of jamu could be due to individuals not being used to the high dosage recommended. In this case, it would be advisable to start on a lower dose so the body gets used to jamu and slowly increase the intake.

Is it harmful to take jamu during menstruation?
No, although it is advisable to avoid taking jamu during this period as it might upset the system.

Is jamu intake addictive?
Certainly not. Once the desired effects are attained, the jamu can be stopped. However, it is wise to take jamu regularly to maintain health.

How does slimming with jamu differ from slimming the Western way?
Western slimming products work like a laxative and reduce fats without providing alternative strength, which results in a haggard look for the slimmer. Jamu slims the natural way. Jamu like Kempes Perut balances your glands and removes old fats but retains the nutritious elements without affecting your appetite or making the skin flabby.

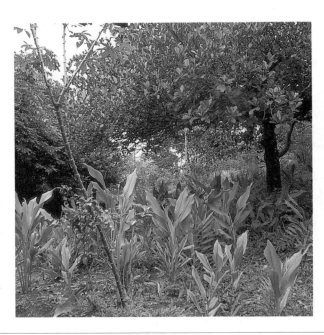

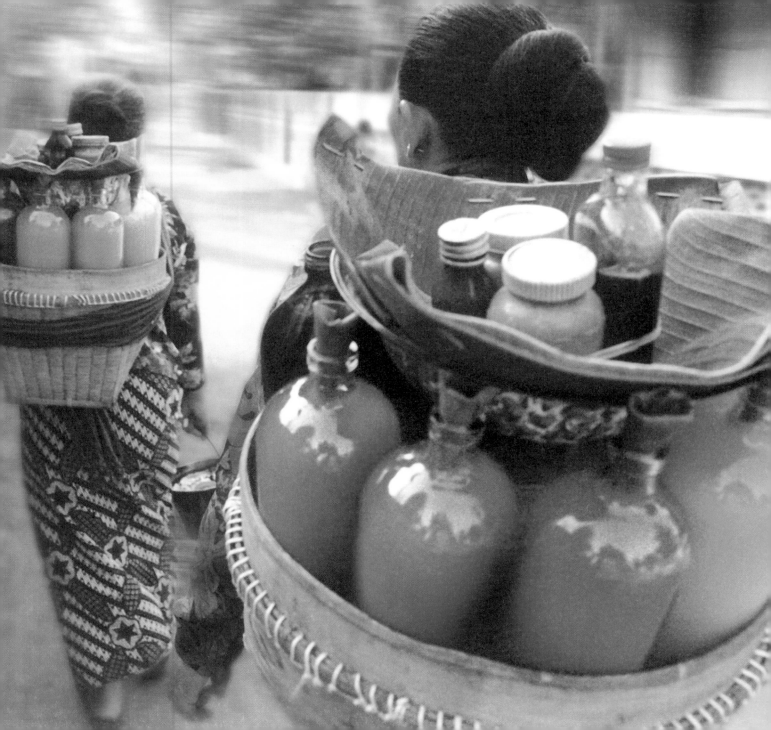

Chapter 2 · Jamu in Daily Life

Despite the diverse range of opinions on this sensitive topic, there is one common perception—the most popular types of jamu enhance and improve sexual performance.

Left:
Jamu gendong *Ibu Nur and her aunt set out at 7 am from her house in Yogyakarta to visit her regular clients.*

So, what exactly is jamu? An easy reply to this question is jamu is Indonesian herbal medicine. But the answer is not that simple, particularly as it is widely believed that jamu is nothing more than a powerful aphrodisiac. Mention jamu in Asia and reactions vary from total dismissal and distrust, to amusement, knowing smiles or perhaps a lengthy discourse on its benefits. Even in Indonesia, people cannot agree on a definition. Everyone knows what jamu is, but each person draws the line in a different place between jamu, medicine and cosmetics. Each jamu may be applied in more than one way; its use depends on the complaint or need. It can be a herbal drink taken to prevent sickness, the answer to chronic illness or an infusion, distillation, brew or paste to treat lifeless hair.

Jamu has also been described as homeopathic medicine. Certainly, there are similarities: both are holistic and plant-based. But the similarity ends there; homeopathy's basic principle of diluting the remedy with upwards of 99 parts alcohol hardly fits with jamu-making techniques or Islamic laws on alcohol. Jamu covers a dazzling array of drinks, pills, capsules and powders said to cure nearly every disease known to man. Indonesian Department of Health officials describes it as "any curing mixture that is taken internally"—certainly a neat definition. Healthcare professionals have their own interpretations, whilst many small-scale producers and even large-scale manufacturers categorize their cosmetics and beauty products as jamu.

Jamu can be used on its own or in conjunction with other healing techniques such as massage. Its advantage is that, if correctly administered, it has no side effects and, according to most Javanese, it is highly effective. Despite the diverse range of opinions on this sensitive topic, there is one common perception—the most popular types of jamu enhance and improve sexual performance.

The Philosophy Behind the Healing

To the outsider, Indonesian herbal medicine appears to be an extremely complex form of healing, combining spiritual, religious, mystical, magical and herbal elements.

Ibu BRA Mooryati Soedibyo, President Director of jamu manufacturer Mustika Ratu and Chairman of the Indonesian Jamu and Traditional Medicine Association tries to summarize it: "Indonesians who believe in God and his powers understand the mythology of jamu in people's lives. God created human beings and provided for their physical health and welfare. According to ecological concepts, nature is meant to prolong life, and life depends on how people use their senses and instincts. Instincts teach us that if there is darkness there must be light; if there is disease there must be a cure; if there is poison there must be an antidote."

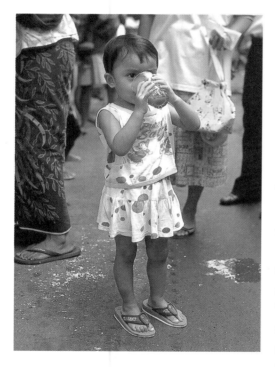

Above:
A girl from a kampung *in south Jakarta drinks her daily dose of jamu.*

The Most Popular Jamu Types

- *Acnarin*, for removing pimples and marks on face; produced by Jamu Indonesia Simona.
- *Antangin*, for the common cold; produced by Deltomed Laboratories.
- *Busterin,* for increasing and beautifying the bust, and for stimulating lactation in breast-feeding mothers; produced by Jamu Indonesia Simona.
- *EM Kapsul*, for women's health and pains in menstruation; produced by Jamu Borobudur.
- *Esha*, to increase spirits and stamina; produced by Jamu Jago.
- *Galian Putri*, for women's all-round health and beauty; produced by Jamu Air Mancur, Nyonya Meneer.
- *Jamu Temu Lawak*, a mild antiseptic wash to help prevent food poisoning; produced by Nyonya Meneer (see below).
- *Kurkumino*, to protect and help the function of the liver; produced by Jamu Ibu.
- *Masuk Angin*, to prevent influenza; produced by Jamu Cap Jago, Jamu Sido Muncul, Nyonya Meneer.
- *Mustika Rapet*, for good sexual health and performance; produced by Jamu Air Mancur.
- *Pegal Linu*, for rheumatism; produced by Jamu Cap Jago, Jamu Air Mancur, Nyonya Meneer, Jamu Sido Muncul, Jamu Sari Ayu.
- *Prolipid*, for reducing cholesterol; produced by Indofarma.
- *Ralinu*, to relieve pain, fatigue and muscle stiffness; produced by Jamu Air Mancur.
- *Sehat Lelaki*, for keeping men in prime form; produced by Jamu Sido Muncul.
- *Susut Perut*, to firm the tummy; produced by Berial Sumber Medica, Jamu Sari Ayu, Mustika Ratu.
- *Wulandari*, a fertility treatment; produced by Jamu Sari Ayu.

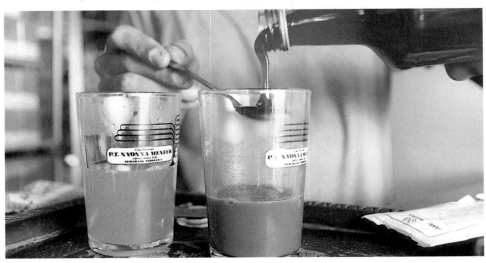

A Jamu Gendong in the Capital City

Thirty-five year old Ibu Jatiatun, or Bu Atun as she is known, is a typical example of a *jamu gendong* working in a large city. She came originally from a small village near Semarang, an area that is famous for its jamu. Because she did not perform well academically, she dropped out of school when she was 10, something she now bitterly regrets. Fortunately, thanks to an aunt who had a fine reputation as a jamu-maker, Bu Atun acquired the basics of jamu.

"From my 65-year-old grandmother to my youngest daughter—we all drink Beras Kencur and Kunir Asem every day and occasionally one of the bitter recipes, and we are very healthy," she announces proudly. "But then my jamu is very safe. All raw materials are boiled before grinding."

"My daughter helps me with the jamu," explains Bu Atun. "We usually make just two kinds and start preparing the night before because I leave on my first round at about 7 am and I'm normally back by 9 am; it takes about two hours to sell everything." Bu Atun makes a second batch of jamu in the afternoon ready for her 4–6 pm sales round in another district.

Although Bu Atun says she never accepts special orders, she does occasionally make a bitter brew from papaya leaves, a concoction which she says is good for flu. "However, it's important to drink lots of water with papaya leaves to counteract the bitterness," she stresses. She also makes Jamu Sirih to treat white vaginal discharge—a problem that affects many women in the tropics from time to time. It's simply a matter of adding betel leaves to the basic Beras Kencur recipe.

Other interesting jamu in Bu Atun's repertoire are Jamu Tujuh Laos, which helps cure rheumatism; Jamu Sehat Wanita recommended for women's health; as well as jamu for amenorrhoea, and a recipe for coughs. She also makes a mix called Cekok, which is produced from a base of Beras Kencur. Although this tastes terrible, it helps small children get back their appetite after an illness.

People who are overweight or women wishing to tighten their stomachs also seek her help. She prepares concoctions from starfruit (*Averrhoa carambola*) for lowering high blood pressure, and other brews to raise it. Bu Atun suggests patients should consult a medical doctor if they are seriously ill, but says many people prefer to take the *jamu gendong*'s advice for such chronic problems as migraine or white discharge.

Since moving to Jakarta, Bu Atun has been able to earn a better living than she would have done if she had stayed in her village. She also sets aside either Thursday or Sunday to perform massage—her grandmother taught her *urut* (see page 100)—which brings in extra money. Although most of the massages are not meant specifically for healing, Bu Atun does perform a special massage for women with sagging or painful wombs which she—and many of her patients—consider very effective.

Considering the substantial weight of a fully laden basket of jamu, I asked how long Bu Atun felt she would—and could—continue this work.

"As long as I'm strong enough, I'll keep going," was her confident reply.

Islam (and Indonesia has the largest Muslim population of any country in the world) embraces the concept that healing the sick is the highest form of service to God. The Qur'an states: "Nature has been created by God for humankind to exploit and use for its good purposes.... God sent down a treatment for every ailment." In this way, both religion and the natural world are harnessed for the making of jamu.

However, even before Islam came to Indonesia in the 14th century, the maintenance of inner and outer harmony was considered essential to good health. Thus, when Islam arrived, it simply reinforced these beliefs. Being ill in the spiritual sense is an ailment for which the average Westerner would not take medicine; but, according to both Javanese and Balinese under-standing of 'health', there are many different 'cures' (just as there are many different causes) for such ailments.

Holistic Approach
Jamu is a holistic therapy. The concept of harmony—balance between a person and their enrionment, or the balance between the hot and cold elements in the body—means that both illness and medicines are divided into hot and cold categories. The herbalist's skill lies in contrasting a hot illness with the appropriate cold medicine and vice versa; hot medicine cures a cold illness and cold mecicine is recommended for a hot illness. Jamu prescriptions always follow this rule, which is why there is a catalogue of antonyms: hot and cold; sweet and sour; bitter and sugary; strong and weak. Similarly, if a formula is developed to treat a specific problem in one organ of the body, the effect on the rest of the system must always be taken into consideration.

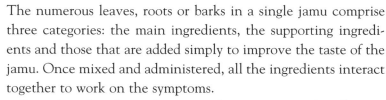

Below:
A well-known jamu shop in Solo that stocks a wide range of different jamu.

The numerous leaves, roots or barks in a single jamu comprise three categories: the main ingredients, the supporting ingredients and those that are added simply to improve the taste of the jamu. Once mixed and administered, all the ingredients interact together to work on the symptoms.

Jamu has four basic functions. It treats particular illnesses (problems as varied as kidney stones, cervical cancer or diarrhoea); it maintains continuing good health (through the promotion of blood circulation and increased metabolism); it relieves aches and pains (by reducing inflammation or by aiding digestive problems); and it also addresses particular malfunctions in the body (such as lack of fertility or unpleasant body odour). Sometimes it can be multi-functional: for example, a jamu may be a general tonic, but it also acts as an antiseptic to prevent stomach infections.

Jamu is not an overnight remedy. Results can only be achieved with regular use over a period of time. And because the 'cure' is gradual, patients do not usually experience any side effects. Some jamu are made from poisonous herbs and if they are not made up and administered correctly, they can be potentially toxic. The herbalist's art lies in knowing how to neutralize these poisonous elements to produce a powerful and curative medicine. Sometimes, jamu will be taken alongside a course of traditional massage to speed up the healing process.

Who Uses Jamu?

Practically every Javanese woman and many Javanese men use jamu on a regular basis. Jamu is recommended for anything from making skin soft and glowing, to producing a tight vagina.

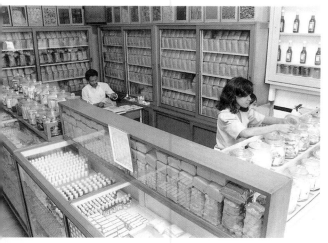

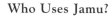

It removes body odour—ask for a deodorant in Java and you are likely to be handed herbal pills. There is jamu for "ensuring harmonious marriage" and one to enhance any number of female charms. A woman is advised to drink Jamu Kamajaya-Kamaratih ('God of Love–Goddess of Love') before marriage in order to "become a housewife loved by her husband". Judging by one copywriter's claim for Jamu Indonesia Simona's Extra Super Venus, no woman should be without it. "It goes without saying that every wife desires her husband's love and attention. But she should also know that every husband desires to see his wife looking fresh, neat, vivacious, healthy, charming and fascinating, even though blessed with many children. If she knows the secret she will not put off taking Extra Super Venus from this moment!"

But not only women swear by jamu: men also worry about their looks and libido, and jamu is widely used to enhance male virility. Indonesian men may well have been amused by the intense publicity given to Viagra, the 1998 'wonder drug' for impotence; they've had their own such remedies for generations. The number of men who queue for their daily dose of Jamu Laki Laki (the 'Man's Medicine', said to keep a man in peak condition) make it one of the most popular drinks. There are pills that promise to "create new energy, man becomes more manly", while another brand professes to change the lives of men who are "sadly lacking in that manly power to perform their part in coitus in spite of the fact that their desires still existed".

The choice of remedies is enormous. There are creams for increasing the size of an erection along with specific directions concerning the massage techniques a woman should use to apply the cream. One helpful taxi driver from Surabaya cheerfully

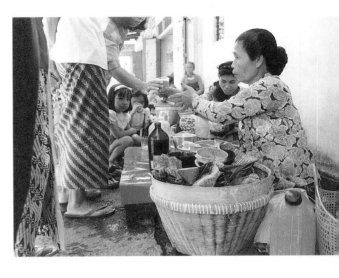

Above:
Wherever you go in Indonesia—in the markets or along the streets—you will see jamu being sold. In Muntilan, near Yogyakarta, a jamu gendong *sells jamu on the side of the pavement.*

How Jamu Works

"The method of (jamu) treatment is very different from the conventional Western approach. In Western medicine drugs usually act to kill an infection, while jamu encourages the body to produce its own antibodies. In other words, jamu acts as a catalyst and does not replace the body's functions. The cure comes from within."
- Part of an interview with Dutch healer, Father Lukman (see page 121).

expanded on this theme to me and explained he personally swore by Kuda-Laut or 'Seahorse Jamu'. Indonesian men also enthusiastically consume jamu to lose weight or to become healthier. Whilst it specializes in enhancing sexual performance, jamu can also cure bloodshot eyes or stiff limbs, reduce hangover headaches, relieve indigestion, stomach upsets, flu, colds and a host of other problems.

However delicately (or bluntly) the notion is expressed, many of these lotions, potions and pills were developed to increase or enhance sexual performance. Why did appearance and sexual attraction become an obsession in Indonesia, an Islamic country where traditional values are extremely strong? The answer may lie in the position that Indonesian men hold in the family unit—one that can assume a quasi-godlike status. This attitude is reinforced by Islamic law, a law that allows men to acquire up to four wives provided they can support them adequately. If a man isn't wealthy (and 80 per cent of the population are not), he will often acquire additional wives before discovering his income cannot cope with the expense. Thus wives can become expendable. In the past, Islam made it relatively easy for men to obtain a divorce and the unlucky wives would be left without a breadwinner, usually with young families to support. Often, the husband simply disappeared to start afresh elsewhere.

Given these circumstances, it's no wonder a wife works hard to hold her husband's attention. Since many men, including Indonesians, usually favour younger girls, the chances of discarded, older wives finding other partners are severely limited. In the past, Indonesian women were raised to accept this situation and turn a blind eye if husbands strayed. This way of life often led to early marriage and informal divorce, and it is still common to find women who have had two or three husbands before the age of 30. With the onus on a wife to keep her man by whatever means, jamu is a formidable ally. For centuries, jamu was made almost exclusively by women, often for women; these specialized herbalists catered to their own female needs and focused the jamu on ways to retain youth and beauty. Indonesian custom dictates that female health and beauty are inextricably bound up with a woman's role as wife and mother, which means sex is a key element in the equation. Naturally, jamu reflects these beliefs and is biased in favour of good health, beauty, marital harmony, sex and large families. Staying attractive was (and often still is) of economic as well as social importance.

Like herbal medicine in other countries, jamu is used mainly as a preventative measure rather than as a cure. It is believed that the various herbs promote good health and purify the blood. Even though some people question their ability to cure, most have their favourite recipe.

Regulating the Industry

The fact that jamu has been empirically, not scientifically, proven has led Indonesian doctors, pharmacists and government health officials to advocate a more scientific approach to the manufacture and prescription of jamu. They insist that claims for herbal medicine must be verified using clinical trials. They also urge that tests must be based on sound pharmacological principles which examine the type, effectiveness, kinetic absorption, metabolism, excretion and the working mechanism of the product, as well as a medicine's therapeutic use. Exhaustive

---

Tips for Jamu Users

Straining the Brew
Some jamu mixtures can leave a residue if not filtered. An example is jamu *godok*, or dried jamu. Instructions normally state that two glasses of water should be added to the dried roots and barks and the mixture boiled till the liquid reduces to one glassful". Then, it should be sieved before it is drunk.

Ibu Hennie's mother had been cheerfully drinking this kind of jamu for years when she was diagnosed as having a gallstone. The doctor told her it was impossible to grind down raw ingredients finely enough in some jamu *godok*; consequently anyone drinking large quantities over a long period could face problems. Liquids pass out of the body whereas residue from the powdered leaves and bark in jamu *godok* remains in the system. In her case the residue had built up and eventually formed a stone.

Refreshing the Mixture for Good Results
Home-made jamu can go bad if it's left lying around too long. To ensure its safety, boil up the mixture again and let the powder sink to the bottom of the saucepan or glass before drinking it.

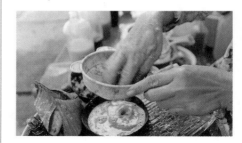

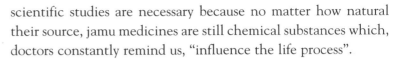

Below:
Jamu basket belonging to jamu gendong *Ibu Sari, containing her daily repertoire. One of the more traditional sellers, Ibu Sari uses banana leaves as bottle stoppers, and only glass (not plastic) bottles. Special orders are wrapped in banana leaves and placed at the top of her basket.*

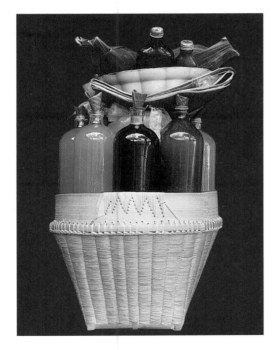

scientific studies are necessary because no matter how natural their source, jamu medicines are still chemical substances which, doctors constantly remind us, "influence the life process".

In 1981, the government set up eight designated herbal medicine testing centres for the development and application of traditional medicine in Java, Sulawesi, Sumatra and Bali. Their brief was the scientific study of commercially manufactured products, with a view to ascertaining whether their healing claims were valid or not. At present, the centres employ two methods of testing. The first deals with the bioactive screening of crude and fractioned extracts. The second, which is called the chemical approach, includes step-by-step experiments that extract, separate, isolate and purify ingredients; the process is technically described as structural elucidation, theoretical deduction of bioactivity and pharmacological testing. It is believed that such trials will bring scientific credibility to a subject that has—up to now—been cloaked in mystery.

Jamu was given further credibility in the late 1980s when an investigative centre opened in Yogyakarta, home of traditional medicine. In answer to popular requests for research and analysis of jamu, Professor Dr Koesnadi Hardjasoemantri, then Director of Gadjah Mada University, set up the Research Centre for Traditional Medicine at the university. The Centre's task is to evaluate traditional medicine, produce experimental batches, train jamu technical staff and develop raw materials. In addition, it now includes massage and acupuncture in its brief. The Centre has also adopted an educational role and operates courses on jamu making in villages throughout Central Java to help small producers improve hygiene and quality.

A Fair Trial

Clinical trials have been implemented in Indonesia, but it is a complex, Herculean task. Not only can a jamu formula consist of 40 or more ingredients, but each may contain a dozen or more chemical components. In addition to the active ingredients, there are secondary, inactive items, used to render the medicine palatable or to mask unpleasant odours. And, as Professor Sutarjadi, founder of Post-Graduate Studies at the University of Airlangga in Surabaya, points out, ingredients from different parts of Java will probably have different properties as soil, climate and altitude differ radically from one area to another.

In terms of manpower and economic resources, the task of analysing and qualifying jamu ingredients and formulæ is colossal. Detractors argue that the industry should not be burdened with such extra requirements when most Indonesians have accepted jamu at face value for centuries. To simplify research, the Indonesian Ministry of Health introduced a new ruling in the late 1990s under the heading 'Phytopharmaca', which loosely translates as 'Active Plant Ingredients'.

This ruling requires that commercial producers reduce complicated formulæ for every curing jamu to five essential ingredients in order to simplify testing. It also requires producers to standardize the active substance in each ingredient. However, a lack of information as to how traditional herbs were originally prepared hinders clarification. The government directive also states that clinical trials for both medical drugs and traditional medicine must be conducted to the same criteria; these are costly at the best of times, all the more so for jamu products which have a comparatively low retail price.

As a concession to this expense, the government has announced that clinical trials may be carried out at Sentra P3T (the Research Centre for the Development and Application of Traditional Treatments) which has the authority to legally authenticate any claims proven during official tests. Although fees for trials here are less expensive than medical drug clinical trials, the cost of this service is still considered beyond most budgets. Results from clinical trials that have been undertaken highlight another important factor of jamu: its versatility. Any one ingredient can be a base ingredient for a formula that addresses a wide range of complaints.

Doctors at Sentra P3T have conducted a number of preliminary clinical trials on selected remedies. The list includes garlic (*bawang putih*; *Allium sativum*) for hypertension; caricature plant (*handeuleum*; *Graptophyllum pictum*) for haemorrhoids; guava leaves (*jambu biji*; *Psidium guajava*) for diarrhoea; round turmeric (*temu lawak*; *Curcuma xanthorrhiza*) for chronic hepatitis and osteoarthritis; cashew nut fruit (*kacang mede*; *Anacardium occidentale*) to reduce pain in acute toothache; and *pare* fruit or bitter gourd (*Momordica charantia*) to treat diabetes mellitus.

The Research Centre for Traditional Medicine in Yogyakarta has also completed the first phase of a study to evaluate the effect of cashew nut leaves in treating rheumatoid arthritis and hypertension. Similar work is being carried out on turmeric (*kunir*; *Curcuma domestica*) and its potential to cure ulcers, and to confirm whether the juice of bitter gourd can help diabetes sufferers. In addition, the research programme is studying dosages, especially as regards Westerners, who may need smaller quantities than people who have taken herbal medicines from birth.

In the early 1990s, the Toray Foundation in Bandung carried out a scientific study to find out whether the very popular product, Pegal Linu (see page 11) had any positive effect on the health of *becak* (trishaw) drivers whose complaints included aches, pains, rheumatics and fatigue. Pegal Linu is composed of, amongst other things, turmeric, ginger, galangal and pepper. The investigating team concluded that it made a substantial difference to the drivers, as it restored energy and reduced muscular pain significantly.

Assuming scientists manage, despite all the obstacles, to complete their experiments and publish their findings, they are more than likely to face a barrage of abuse from the various jamu companies who protest that competitors will steal the formulæ if results list chemical components. Yet, notwithstanding all these difficulties, the government continues with its testing programmes, owing to an increasing awareness of the export potential of the country's myriad jamu products.

The Professional Viewpoint

For Indonesians, Western medicine is a recent and expensive phenomenon. Not only are allopathic drugs and ointments well beyond the pocket of the average Indonesian, but they are not a tempting alternative to jamu which has been used successfully for generations.

Although there are detractors who consider herbal medicine ineffective, jamu is gaining ground. There is no doubt that jamu mixtures are full of active, natural ingredients such as vitamins A, C and E, all of which contribute to overall well-being. Indeed many of the barks, leaves, roots, stems, flowers, seeds and

Ibu Risma and the Rosy Periwinkle

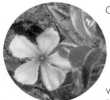

Cancer is a fast-growing disease in Indonesia with over 190,000 new patients recorded each year. Twenty-eight year old Risma Abednego was told she had cancer, a fist-sized tumour in her womb, and her only chance was an operation—one she rejected. She was encouraged to seek out Bapak Soetijono Darsosentono, a traditional healer in Yogyakarta, who specialized in curing cancer.

He gave her traditional medicine consisting of dried *benalu* (*Loranthes* sp.) and *tapak dara* (rosy or Madagascar periwinkle; *Catharanthus roseus*) leaves. He told her to clean the leaves, boil them and drink the water. She was to repeat the process with betel nut leaves. Smoking, drinking, and the consumption of preserved, instant, spicy and sour foods, as well as lamb and seafood, were all banned. For nine months, Risma consumed large amounts of soya in the form of tempe or tofu, before returning to her doctor for a check-up. He noticed a great improvement. Eighteen months later he pronounced her completely cured.

Patients treated by Bapak Soetijono Darsosentono are urged to continue taking the medicine every day for five years. Risma developed cancer over 10 years ago but still drinks the healing brew as an insurance policy and everyone in the house follows her healthy diet. Not surprisingly, she has become an enthusiastic supporter of traditional medicine.

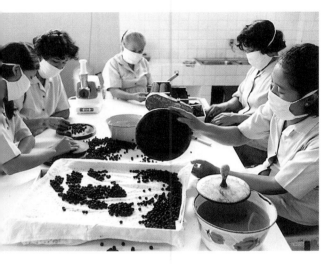

Above:
The factory that produces one of the country's best-selling jamu, Posodolamatee. Government regulations are beginning to standardize production in such businesses.

minerals used come straight from the country's tropical rainforests, where there is no pollution or pesticides and hence are at their purest and most potent.

The accusation that jamu is 'not scientifically proven' is still often made by the medical profession. Perhaps it is not proven in the same terms as we expect from Western medicine, but the results speak for themselves. The medical profession should note that without the benefit of expensive modern products, Javanese women are amazingly well preserved despite having given birth to large families. Unlike their Western counterparts, who often remain overweight after giving birth, Indonesian mothers soon regain their pre-pregnancy form. They take a course of jamu, after-birth massage and binding, and will use up to ten different jamu formulæ internally and externally for 40 days to cleanse the body, contract the muscles, lose weight, or—as instructions on one after-birth jamu pack state—"restore vigour and reinforce sex appeal". Six weeks later, these women are back in pre-pregnancy shape. How many Western women can say the same after the birth of a child?

As we have noted, the Indonesian Government has been instrumental in persuading the medical profession to consider jamu seriously and research the range of products. Among these professionals, there are many doctors, both Western and Indonesian-trained, who never go without their daily potion of jamu. Admitting it is another matter. Many consume herbal drinks in secret because they feel that endorsing jamu does not sit well with their image as modern, medical practitioners. Modern-thinking patients might lose faith in their doctor if they had the slightest notion he believed in jamu. There are doctors, however, that recognize the efficacy of traditional medicine and prescribe jamu herbs without disclosing that fact to their patients. These pills are not supplied by recognized jamu makers but made on prescription at the local pharmacy; these concoctions include popular and successful jamu ingredients (such as turmeric or ginger).

Acceptance by Westerners

Until recently, most Westerners have been cautious about using jamu. Some are afraid that medicines produced in a developing country may not be safe or hygienic. Up to now such details as methods, dosage and active ingredients have been irrelevant to villagers who have used jamu for centuries: jamu cures—that is all they need to know. But the producers of jamu want to go beyond the villages, and even beyond the borders of the country.

Now that the government has imposed clinical trials and has set up research centres, it is believed that attitudes to traditional medicine will change. After all, any inexpensive system of medicine that purports to solve any problem, from curing arthritis or frigidity, hypertension or cancer, to improving fertility or regulating the appetite, improving the hair and helping a teenage girl adjust to puberty, is worth investigating on all levels. Jamu's reputation has already turned it into an important export to the Netherlands, but figures have only touched on what is destined to become a vast industry. It is no accident that the herbs used in Indonesian preparations frequently form the basis of many Western medicines, and it is no coincidence that Anita Roddick, founder of Bodyshop, spent many years researching for her health and beauty products in Indonesia.

Choosing Ingredients

Traditionally Indonesian jamu was made on a daily basis by the women of the house. This was essential before refrigeration and the habit has stuck. The quality of the ingredients plays as important a part in producing effective jamu as their freshness. Even today, an Indonesian housewife may take a quick stroll round her garden to collect the extra jamu ingredients she cannot find in the market or the ones she needs in minuscule amounts. She believes home-made is best, insisting that many sellers cut cost by skimping on expensive, active ingredients like the rhizome of *kencur* (resurrection lily; *Kaempferia galanga*).

Whether her recipes are passed down through the family or are derived from books, there is a degree of elasticity in all the formulæ and measuring ingredients can vary. Some recipes state the number of *ons* (equivalent to 100 g); another method is to state the amount in terms of 'fingers, a thumb or a handful'; yet others state quantities by price (Rp 200 betel leaf, Rp 100 sugar and so on). This is fairly haphazard unless you know the price of herbs when the book was written, and particularly so since the drastic devaluation of the currency in 1997/98. However, most Indonesians are familiar with the vagaries of the terminology and have learned through experience.

While the simplicity of jamu-making is often stressed—after all, what is easier than mixing up an effective cure from ingredients growing in the garden—it is, in reality, complex and has many pitfalls. Recipes and ingredients appear deceptively easy to the newcomer, keen to experiment. First-timers would be advised to enlist the aid of either a jamu seller or a herbalist, or simply take the remedies rather than try to make them.

For instance, sugar is an important base ingredient in many healing recipes. Indonesian jamu is made from three types of sugar. *Gula batu* (rock sugar; *Saccharum officinarum*) is refined white sugar. *Gula Jawa* or *gula merah* (coconut sugar; *Cocos nucifera*) is made from the sap of young coconut trees and cooked at high temperatures to produce its brown colour. The syrup is left to cool and harden in empty coconut shells and assumes the discus-like shape. The third variety, *gula Aren* (palm sugar), is the queen of sugars, made from the pure sap of a young Aren tree (*Arenga pinnata*). Its colour changes from white to brown during cooking and the solid sugar is shaped into small cylinders before it reaches shops and market stalls. This sugar is the most expensive of the three, but many women refuse to settle for anything less, for they say the cheaper types of sugar affect the taste and quality of their jamu. This criticism is sometimes levelled at *jamu gendong* (herbal tonic street sellers) who often substitute a factory-made synthetic similar to saccharin, which is said to cause coughs.

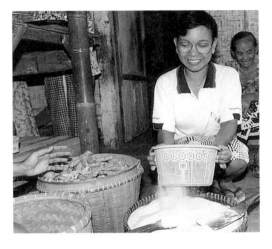

More problems may arise for the jamu novice with the simplification of common names in Indonesia. For example, the ingredients *manis jangan*, *kayu manis* and *kayu legi* all translate into English as 'sweet wood' but each is different botanically. *Kayu manis* (*Cinnamomum zeylanicum*) and *manis jangan* (*Cinnamomum burmanii*) are respectively the Indonesian and Javanese names for the sweet-tasting wood we know in the West as cinnamon: both are used in jamu. However, *kayu legi* is Javanese for a sweet bark that has no flavour, is brown outside, white in the centre and is used for general cooking (Chinese liquorice; *Glycyrrhiza glabra*).

Above:
The quality of the ingredients is key to good jamu. This jamu maker always strains sugar before use; on left is a basket of fresh turmeric.

Fresh Jamu

Many Indonesians will drink jamu only in the form of finely chopped herbs, or powder mixed with water, because these are deemed closest to the natural herbal state and therefore more effective. For these adepts, traditional medicine in a pre-packed, ready-to-swallow form holds no attraction. They put up with the inconvenience of making these mixtures and accept their often bitter, unpalatable taste. The reluctant jamu taker will find that adding a pinch of salt to the glass lessens the shock to the taste-buds. A slice of lemon or a little honey is also recommended. Sieving the jamu through muslin gets rid of the indigestible, floating remains. A seasoned jamu drinker will down a glass in one, which reduces exposure to the, frankly, often disgusting taste. Eating a piece of fruit, especially a banana or papaya, is suggested to remove the aftertaste. Fresh and natural are the key words in these preparations.

Commercial growth, however, has meant these old ways are not always practical, especially for city dwellers. To meet the demands of the urban market, larger producers process over 700 tons of ingredients into jamu pills and capsules each month. Modern manufacturing methods enable factories to produce sufficient quantities to make export a possibility. And while reluctance by the old school to share health and beauty secrets with outsiders hampered the industry in its infancy, this problem has now been overcome by the pressures of an expanding economy. The lure of overseas markets is proving stronger than the mysticism that once surrounded jamu. If the end product has a longer shelf life, the horizons for export are limitless.

Choosing and Drinking Jamu

Whatever one's needs, jamu can almost certainly supply an answer, but it may require experimentation to find the right manufacturer. Pegal Linu, for instance, concocted by one manufacturer to counteract rheumatism and tiredness, may make no difference to symptoms, whilst the same medicine produced by another company could bring instant relief. Experimentation with products from different companies is often necessary. Furthermore, manufacturers warn that jamu works slowly, on the basis of the body's self-healing capabilities, and it may take up to two months before results are noticed.

Then there is the problem of how to take the potion. Jamu is steeped in folklore that is respected but rarely explained. For example, why is jamu drunk standing up straight with one's big toes crossed? Few people know the answer: most can only reply that it is tradition. Yet they still do it! One school of thought insists that jamu must be drunk facing the sun. This accords with the principles relating to spiritual energy, where the sun is a symbol of light and divine power, representing the oneness of everything. On a more pragmatic level, the sun warms the body, automatically relaxing the muscles and enabling the body's systems to absorb the herbs more efficiently.

Herbalists warn never to drink jamu with alcohol because the latter dissolves the jamu, thus cancelling out its benefits. Furthermore, freshly ground roots and powders may sink to the bottom of a glass and end up being washed down the sink: the solution is to stir and drink the mixture immediately. To make jamu more potent, some advise whisking in a fresh chicken or quail egg (but not duck or turtle eggs). This is a popular addition

A Glossary of Common Indonesian Terms

air • water

arang • charcoal

Bapak (or Pak) • polite form of address for an elder man

daun • leaf

dukun • healer/traditional doctor

gula • sugar

Ibu (or Bu) • polite form of address for a woman

jamu gendong • jamu seller

kampung • village

kraton • palace

minyak • oil

nasi • cooked rice

obat • medicine

pasar • market

pisang • banana

pilis • compress

toko • shop

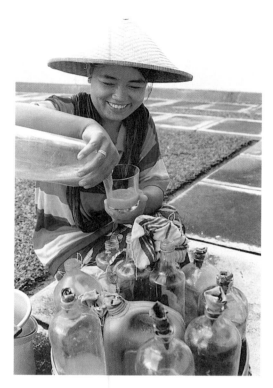

Above:
Jamu gendong *in
Solo pouring Kunir
Asem into a glass.
Jamu is usually sold
twice a day, in the
early mornings and
again in the late after-
noon when people are
on their way home.*

to many powdered jamu and is normally mixed into Jamu Cabe Puyang (an abbreviation of *cabe jawa*, the fruit of *Piper retrofractum*, a type of pepper, and *lempuyang pahit*, the rhizome of the bitter ginger, *Zingiber amaricans*). Jamu Cabe Puyang is often prescribed for people who are run down.

The right *jamu gendong* or seller is the best route to successful jamu taking. It is expected that the *jamu gendong* will pose a number of questions to ascertain whether an ailment might be related to other complaints, due to pregnancy, vaccinations, and so on, and therefore will have a better idea which jamu is most suitable. A lack of experience can lead to the wrong mixture which, not surprisingly, will not work.

Rituals that Govern Jamu

As with many traditions, jamu has its fair share of superstitions that must be addressed to eliminate potential dangers or to ensure the healing properties of the medicine. Many of these beliefs stem from practical considerations: some are long since lost, others are easier to recognize. It is not just a question of adding an extra ingredient or the angle you face when taking a potion: it is what might happen if you do not. For instance, it is believed that if a woman breaks her grinding stone, disaster will befall her household. To prevent this, she must then walk around the house, naked, seven times. For the Javanese house-hold, jamu is vital and if a wife breaks her tools, there is no way to protect against ills. Likewise, no self-respecting housewife will leave her pestle and mortar on the doorstep because her husband, coming home after a day's work in the rice fields, could trip over it, break his neck and be unable to support his family.

Another superstition states that quantities of an ingredient have to be twice "the number of the day when born". This presents an unusual problem nowadays as the Javanese calendar is based on the five-day week. The normal seven-day week is made to fit into this by simple addition. For example, a Javanese woman would understand that if she was born on Saturday Pahing 9, and the recipe called for twice that amount, she has to add 18 ingredients to a recipe. Conflicting with this is the superstition that ingredients must be of an odd number. Thus you may include one or three handfuls of an ingredient, or one or five cups of liquid, but never two. Some recipes for jamu furthermore require the preparation of the medicine by a girl who has yet to start menstruating—yet another hurdle.

Other beliefs concern the need for additional ingredients for pregnant women. They are advised to include the powdered egg shells of newly-hatched, healthy chickens and carbonized mouse nests in their jamu. The egg shells are included in the hope that the baby will be equally healthy; they provide additional calcium while the carbon helps absorb toxins. The mouse nests were believed to make birthing as easy as that of a mouse.

Jamu also features in Javanese wedding ceremonies in which the bride's mother presents a newly married couple with a box or *botekan* containing various seeds, rhizomes and dried cuttings from traditional medicinal plants and spices. Traditionally, these should be used on the first day of marriage and, more importantly, be planted in the garden of the couple's new home. This gesture is a mother's last symbolic effort to provide a healthy life for her daughter.

A Cautionary Tale

It is vital to follow instructions when mixing jamu. Barbara Johnson, an American who has lived in Jakarta for many years, discovered this at her own expense. Although Barbara has a fine figure she noticed the beginnings of cellulite on the back of her thighs. Mentioning this to an Indonesian friend, she was amazed when a pack of dried roots and herbs arrived at her house a few days later. "This is for the cellulite," her friend said. "I've used it for years and it works wonders."

Barbara asked her maids, village girls with experience of jamu, to prepare the drink and promptly forgot about it. She later found a glass of black liquid in the fridge and, enquiring what it was, learned that it was her jamu. Naturally she was keen to see whether this foul-tasting brew was effective and drank it all down only to realize minutes later that she'd made a big mistake.

Barbara was rushed to hospital, having burned her throat, oesophagus and intestines to such an extent that she couldn't go home for six weeks. She says the only good part of this tale was the result. "When I looked in the mirror I discovered there was not one single ounce of cellulite anywhere on my body. The cure was incredible in more ways than one."

Why did this happen? Apparently Barbara had consumed about three weeks' supply of jamu in one draught, because the girls had accidentally made the mixture far too strong.

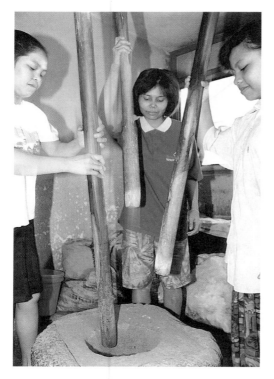

Old beliefs are not in short supply. Some believed that ingredients had to be ground in the home of the person drinking the jamu. However, if that person did not possess a grinding stone, the jamu maker had to decide whether it was appropriate to make the jamu in his or her own home before delivering it to the client. It was also considered part of the cure for the jamu maker to give the jamu directly to the recipient. If it was a paste, the maker would clean the grinding stone with her hands, and then rub a little of the mixture onto the patient's skin. If the medicine was to be drunk, the jamu maker would put a little of the ground mixture into the glass of jamu with her fingers before the patient was allowed to take it.

Government Regulations

In the interests of safety, the government advises that only those brands of jamu carrying the Indonesian Food and Drug Control Directorate (the DepKes RI number) on the packet should be consumed. (DepKes is the acronym for the Departemen Kesehatan, the Department of Health and RI stands for Republic of Indonesia.) These registration numbers (issued also by the Departemen Kesehatan) must, by law, be printed on every bottle or packet. The number is issued only after the product has been tested by government laboratories and met a stringent set of requirements. If the name or formula of the jamu changes after registration the whole process must be repeated.

The Department of Health regularly buys herbal medicine from retail outlets to verify that products are not sold after their expiry date and then submits these samples for testing by its team of pharmacists to ensure standards of quality control and

Above:
Large mortars such as these would normally be used by small businesses, whereas smaller versions are used in a normal household.

storage conditions have been met. Some smaller producers, however, simply cannot afford to pay the DepKes registration fees but still make excellent jamu. In this instance a specialist jamu shop should be able to offer advice.

The government now insists every jamu and herbal medicine company employs a qualified pharmacist (or assistant pharmacist) to ensure professional quality control. It has laid down that the word jamu and not *obat* (which means any type of medicine, either natural, as in jamu, or chemical) must be printed on packages of anything that has not been scientifically and clinically tested. In addition, manufacturers are not allowed to advertise that a certain illness can be cured by a specific manufactured jamu. An example of this policy concerns a Slimming Tea. Not only have customers successfully lost weight using this jamu, but it has been scientifically proven that it reduces cholesterol levels too. However, government regulations prevent manufacturers from publicizing this because the product is categorized as jamu, not *obat*.

DepKes regulations stipulate pharmaceutical and medical terminology cannot be used to describe the use and effectiveness of jamu. Any claims on behalf of the product must be in simple, everyday language. Generally, an interval of at least one hour, if not four hours, should separate the consumption of more than one type of jamu.

A Question of Authenticity

As a general rule, it is better to stick with reputable brand names unless the person making up the medicine has been recommended as entirely trustworthy. There are extremely good

Below:
At Kabupaten it is thought the villagers have a special relationship with jamu. The village is dominated by an imposing statue of a soldier and a jamu seller to commemorate the revolution. The inscription draws attention to jamu's role in the struggle: "If you take our land you will be killed, Even if we die defending it. If the people are healthy, the country is strong."

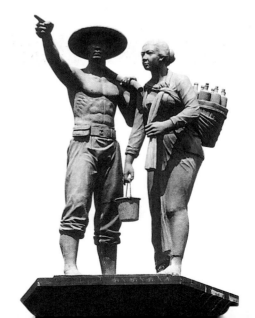

healers who do not have the advantage of scientific staff and machinery, but one needs to be sure they really are experts. There are stories of manufacturers who have added a hefty dose of steroids to the concoction. The result may be effective in the short term but it certainly is not safe. A guarded approach is essential, because it is easy to pick someone who is a charlatan.

Another area for concern is the proliferation of one type of night *warung*, small stalls that usually stay open all night in Indonesia. Illegal jamu is big business. The sellers are well known to locals in Bali or Yogyakarta and are occasionally found in Jakarta. As their products are illegal, these traders are expert at uprooting themselves and disappearing at the first sign of police. If undisturbed, they make an extremely good living and the benefits outweigh the risks. However, they sell an exceedingly strong jamu that can be highly dangerous. It is similar to a fermented wine or beer and is famous, according to Indonesians, for 'making men strong'. It is one of the few jamu with side effects. If you notice a group of men reeling and singing around a night stall, chances are they have been working on their virility because the fermented drink makes customers exceedingly drunk. Foreigners do not have to worry about stumbling across these sellers because they would never let a Westerner buy their jamu. They are equally reluctant to sell to an Indonesian woman who arrives on her own, but will serve her if she is with her husband.

There are also more or less legitimate sellers who think they can improve on original recipes. One such vendor in Menteng Dalam, North Jakarta has a reputation for selling exceedingly good jamu made using an electric blender; he attracts huge queues of regular customers in the morning rush hour. What is

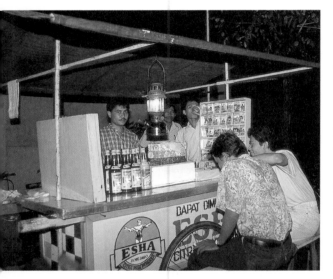

Above:
Jakarta is a city that never sleeps and some highly reputable jamu stalls stay open all night to cater to customer needs. One such stall is shown here.

so unique about this jamu? The seller adds a Bodrex tablet (a trade name for paracetamol) to the blender with every glass of jamu even though it is illegal to mix jamu with chemical drugs. On its own, this is not such a bad thing as many Western doctors recommend a small dosage of paracetamol each day. The real problem is that good jamu is so carefully concocted that if it is tampered with, toxic chemical reactions are liable to occur.

Pharmacists on the staff of Indonesia's major cosmetic and herbal medicine manufacturers warn against jamu that is not stored properly. When jamu becomes damp, perfect conditions exist for poisonous fungi to develop in the bottle or packet. For this reason, manufacturers seal their packets and bottles thoroughly and instruct retailers not to exceed the sell-by dates.

Currently there is no systematic approach to traditional medicine in Indonesia, which is why manufacturer Martina Berto has set up scientific procedures to standardize jamu at every stage of research and production. Before launching a new product, the research and development staff test the jamu by taking the recommended dose themselves. It will only be launched if no negative physiological effects result. In addition, they carry out efficacy as well as toxicity studies (including acute and sub-acute toxicity studies) and the product is carefully monitored once it enters the marketplace. They are not alone in moving towards more stringent regulations: major competitors such as Nyonya Meneer have also instigated quality controls that inspire confidence. There are charlatans in any country and the Indonesian Jamu Association constantly warns the public against using illegally manufactured products and advises buying exclusively from the 500 brands on its own register.

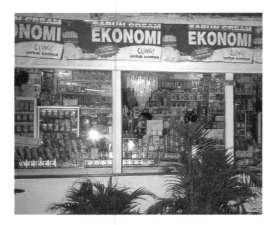

Traditional Healthcare Elsewhere in Indonesia

It could be argued if you understand Javanese jamu, there is no need for further research into the subject because the range and sophistication of Javanese traditional remedies covers the entire spectrum of Indonesian healing. Although most Indonesians, and especially the Javanese, would support this hypothesis, the archipelago is home to many different approaches to healthcare. Such variations are mainly due to the type of plants and trees growing in a particular region and their accessibility. For example, in 1977 a research team in Kendari, Southeast Sulawesi, found 449 herbal remedies still being used, and this excluded dozens of unpatented herbal mixtures known only to the locals.

Kalimantan

Kalimantan in Javanese means 'River of Diamonds', but these provinces on the island of Borneo actually get their name from *lamanta* or sago starch, the local staple. Home to the giant Rafflesia plant that can grow up to one metre in diameter, the island's diverse geography, rainfall and temperature make it one of the richest biodiversities in the world. The original inhabitants turned this living apothecary to advantage by learning which plants and trees had healing properties. Medical treatments were a combination of charms, magic, ritual and herbs. A recent study showed that while some tribes relied on as few as 12 medicinal plants, others were using up to 213 different species.

Nutmeg (*Myristica fragrans*), indigenous to the Moluccas (Maluku), is one of Indonesia's most famous trees. In Europe, it is primarily valued as a spice; in Kalimantan, it is regarded as a medicine. The mace or lacy covering of the nutmeg seed can

Above:
A small jamu shop in south Jakarta which is open till late at night and features a chandelier as part of its interior design.

A Change of Career and Change in Fortunes

An educated woman, Ibu Sri is forty-two years old and has sold jamu for the past five years. She started life as an elementary school teacher but couldn't manage on such a small salary. After various unsatisfactory jobs, Ibu Sri worked her way through books on jamu making and experimented for over a year until she was satisfied with the results. Because these were cures for serious illness as opposed to recipes to keep the body healthy, she verified the complicated formulæ with her cousin, a doctor, to be sure the mixtures were safe.

Like most Central Javanese, Ibu Sri grew up with herbal medicine but received a rather special training. She lived with her grandmother at the *kraton* until she was 25, long enough to receive a thorough grounding in the palace herbal medicine. "I use her recipes but you'll never find them in books: things like treating diarrhoea, making face powder, caring for hair and ingredients to make skin smooth."

The children help their mother after school. Unemployed, her husband helps out too, although he has difficulty understanding the jamu formulæ. This means his assistance is limited but he does occasionally buy ingredients when he cycles to the market in Yogyakarta.

Ibu Sri's set up is unusual because she claims to cure 35 ailments including diarrhoea, dysentery, food poisoning and cancer. Remedies for asthma and tiredness, and medicines to prevent or cure female complaints are among her best sellers.

While unaware of the scientific data, Ibu Sri has a fair idea of the chemical action of her ingredients. Customers generally tell her their symptoms, which enables her to choose the most suitable jamu for them. "We mustn't forget that jamu was the forerunner of modern pharmacy and widely used before anyone dreamt of synthetic drugs," she admonishes. "I believe my own family has kept healthy thanks to jamu. It was effective hundreds of years ago and it's effective now."

This maker knows most formulæ by heart but if memory fails Ibu Sri checks the details in a well-thumbed exercise book. Everything is written by hand in Old Javanese and amended with improvements to the original formulæ. Because the research was painstakingly long, she keeps the formulæ secret and the recipes will pass on to her family only on her death.

She is proud her jamu keeps people healthy and can cure serious illness but she also spoke enthusiastically about her potions that can be used to lengthen and condition the hair—a good illustration of the blurred boundary between health and beauty care.

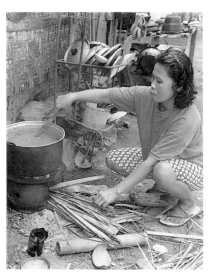

How does Ibu Sri see herself? "I'm a healer starting out as a business-woman." What does she see as her greatest problem? "My hands," came the unexpected response, "They become very sore from the heavy work. I do everything manually you see—crushing, mixing and cooking." Old-fashioned tools for making pills or turning mixtures into powder don't help. Ibu doesn't even use weighing scales to measure the ingredients—she doesn't own a set and relies on spoons instead.

"I can't complain really," she said, "I'm thankful I'm strong and healthy enough to cope with the work. Besides, in my business I can't admit to being sick, can I?"

banish headaches and, when dried, the flowers are often added to jamu recipes. The bark and leaves contain essential oil and different parts of the plant are variously used as an aphrodisiac, a cure for diarrhoea, a purgative or a gargle. Carrying a nutmeg is said to be good for muscular aches, pains and rheumatism. When cut, the bark of the nutmeg tree oozes with a watery, pink sap that dries to the colour of blood, hence its Malay name, *pendarah* (blood). This has strong, magical connotations in Indonesia and is frequently used to describe the kris, a dagger said to possess magic powers.

Another commonly used plant is *Strychnos ignatii* from the Strychnine family. Its local name is *bidara laut* (sea tree), but perversely, it is found in the mountains and forests. An infusion of the root bark is considered a wonderful tonic. Steeped in a glass of water, *bidara laut* stimulates the appetite, cures indigestion, diarrhoea and fatigue, as well as hundreds of other ills.

Maternity care in Kalimantan is surprisingly effective. The expectant mother is given an oil to rub over the stomach during the last two months of pregnancy. Immediately before the birth, she takes a drink that ensures labour rarely lasts longer than 15 minutes. Many Western women would pay a fortune for such an express delivery, but the secrecy surrounding this medicine means it will probably never happen. A shrub with dark red wood, needle-like leaves and the smell of lavender grows in the fallow grassy areas of the island. It is called *ujung atap* (roof edge; *Baeckea frutescens*) and has a multitude of uses, including encouraging menstruation and abortion, and is also a diuretic. Mixed with water, it is drunk for abdominal pain and features strongly in medicines taken after childbirth.

A quick look at medicine used in Kalimantan shows that barks account for three-quarters of the ingredients. One bottle contained eight different materials and was recommended for an astonishing total of 32 ailments from backache and poisoning to impotence and syphilis. One can only assume the concoction works on the principle of normalizing the body functions, curing everything in its path.

Camphor trees (*Pluchea balsamifera* or *Drybalanops aromatica*) are a lucrative business in rainforests, but because many of the trees are scattered, they are not worth tapping. However, a good tree can produce six to seven kilos of resin and a handsome reward for the finder. The precious liquid is used to stimulate heart and blood circulation, and is also accepted in Western medicine as a mild antiseptic and anaesthetic.

By far the most popular plants to emerge from the forests of East Kalimantan are *pasak bumi* (peg of the earth; *Eurycoma longifolia*) and its partner, *tabat barito* (Borneo fig; *Ficus deltoidea*). *Pasak bumi* is also called *bidara laut*, so its Latin name, *Eurycoma longifolia*, is often used to avoid confusion with the genuine *bidara laut* (see left). The root bark—very bitter—is reputed to be one of nature's most powerful male aphrodisiacs. *Tabat barito* has the same effect on women and is an important ingredient in female Love Herb tablets. Their combined use is said to be earth shattering! Sadly, unless someone mounts a rescue operation soon, such experiences are on the wane because both plant species are classified as endangered.

With at least 4,000 species of plants found in Kalimantan, its rainforests have enormous potential for new medicines. However, excessive logging, slash-and-burn farming methods

Below:
*Basic ingredients for
Kunir Asem being
ground with a* pipisan
and gandik, *essential
tools in the kitchen.*

and spontaneous forest fires mean these riches could well be lost forever, unless projects such as Barito Ulu (see page 94) receive adequate funding before it is too late.

The Moluccas

Ceram in Maluku has a reputation for magic, but the use of herbs is also paramount, as a research team discovered in 1980 when they listed 30 species of medicinal plants commonly used on Ceram. The remedies are made from the indigenous leaves, roots and barks, and used for ailments ranging from cough, diarrhoea, fever and backache, to wart removal, swelling, itchiness and bruises. Here, as elsewhere in the Moluccas, all medicines are reserved for serious illness and administered only when symptoms appear. This totally contrasts with the Javanese concept of prevention, body maintenance and ongoing beauty care.

Until recently, the majority of modern, educated Moluccans chose Western medicines, provided they were available and affordable; they resorted to folk medicine only when Western methods did not produce results. Nowadays, many islanders are deciding that synthetic ingredients in modern drugs often make them feel worse instead of better. Western flu medicine, which can make a patient sleepy, is an example, whereas alternative medicine for flu does not produce unpleasant side effects. Moluccans are increasingly turning to traditional methods. Gathering barks, roots and leaves is easy, and costs are low because raw materials are picked from the garden or countryside. Making up formulæ is not a chore either, as locals simply mix the leaves with oil or water, then squeeze them into small round pills. The pills do not last long, as people take the medicine until

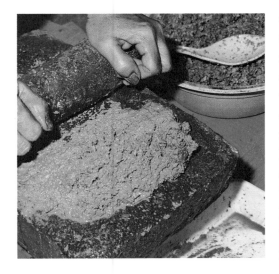

they feel better, then stop. Families in remote villages favour these old-fashioned cures; for many, there is no alternative.

Unfortunately, much of the ancient healing knowledge has been lost. However, the village of Mamala practices an old Muslim custom that illustrates the curing properties of their oil. Each year, seven days after Idul Fitri (the celebration marking the end of the fasting month), a volunteer is whipped on the back and shoulders with sharply-edged palms from the *aren* or sugar palm tree. This continues till the skin is bleeding and raw. When the ordeal is over, the victim's skin is rubbed with a special oil that heals it within 24 hours. The oil, appropriately called Minyak Mamala (Mamala oil), is made only at Idul Fitri, but can be used throughout the year. This is why there is an annual influx of *dukun patah tulang*, bone masseurs and manipulators, who descend on the village to buy stocks for the next 12 months.

Sumatra

For centuries, Sumatra has had its own alternative medicine known as *tambar*. According to one Sumatran pharmacist, these medicines contain herbs and animal products, especially birds. These products usually contain coconut oil as well, which turns them rancid within a week, adding an obnoxious smell. Magic is also sometimes involved in curing. Medicines in Aceh are mixed to a dough-like consistency using a mixture of herbs, animal products and coconut oil; they are kneaded and then rolled into small, brown balls and used for improving strength and blood circulation. The pills have such a good reputation that Malaysia has been importing large quantities for years, despite the fact that it manufactures its own jamu.

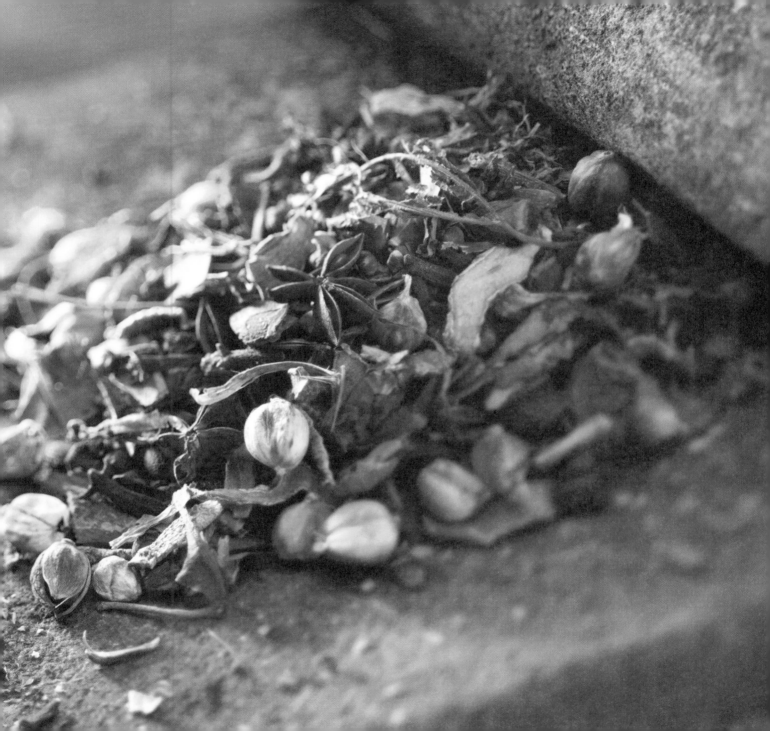

Chapter 3. The Raw Ingredients of Jamu

Despite the large number of plants available, only a handful of species are the undisputed superstars of jamu—they all belong to the ginger or Zingeberaceae family.

Of the 40,000 species of tropical plants in the world, an estimated 30,000 grow in Indonesia. The archipelago is one of the most biodiverse regions in the world. To date, some 7,000 cultivated species have been identified. Close to 1,000 of these are commonly used in the preparation of Indonesia's traditional medicine, although only 286 plants have been registered in the Materia Medika Indonesia at the Department of Health.

This last figure reflects those species used by the major jamu producers, who struggle to keep 200 essential ingredients in stock at any one time. Jamu sellers working from home use up to 100 plants on an ad hoc basis, but focus on only 10 or 12 when preparing their daily stocks. The balance of 700 to 800 plants is used by villagers for a vast range of formulæ that never appear in official records. By contrast, the Ministry of Agriculture maintains that the industry needs no more than 20 medicinal plants.

Over the centuries, Indonesians have experimented with their botanical heritage in numerous ways. There is no doubt that huge number of medicinal plants were selected for their effective healing powers; others may have been used because of

Left:
Raw materials about to go under the gandik *or grinding stone for the first crushing.*

similarities between the characteristics of the plant and the ailment, as dictated by the popular doctrine of signatures or similarities. This suggests that the shape, colour or texture of each plant is a sign virtually telling us what ailments it can cure. Thus, hair-like plants are supposed to make hair grow, flowers with eyes give sharper vision, heart-shaped leaves cure heart disease, red blooms are effective against bleeding, while orchids are excellent aphrodisiacs.

Despite the large number of plants available, only a handful of species are the undisputed superstars of jamu. They all belong to the ginger or Zingiberaceae family: turmeric (*kunir*; *Curcuma domestica*); greater galangal (*lengkuas*; *Languas galanga*); resurrection lily (*kencur*; *Kaempferia galanga*); *lempuyang pahit* (bitter ginger; *Zingiber amaricans*); *lempuyang wangi* (*Zingiber aromaticum*) and *temu lawak* (*Curcuma xanthorrhiza*) (neither of which have common English names) and, of course, common ginger (*jahe*; *Zingiber officinale*). These members of the ginger family are the mainstays of jamu, used both for cosmetics and traditional medicine.

The Ginger Family
Outside Asia, ginger is usually thought to be just the one rhizome, which is used primarily for culinary purposes. The name actually applies to a whole family of rhizomes, Zingiberaceae, with around 200 species recorded so far in Indonesia. These rhizomes are different in shape, colour, flavour and curing ability. Many of these gingers feature on the World Health Organization (WHO) list of the most popular medicinal plants used in 23 countries.

An amazing number of different jamu are created using various combinations of certain basic gingers. Typically this involves grinding the ginger rhizome into a fine paste to which other types of plants are added for their cumulative effect. Once they are mixed together, a chemical reaction is set up that changes a jamu's healing power and substantially increases the gamut of cures.

Common ginger (*jahe; Zingiber officinale*)

The best known member of the Zingiberaceae family, common ginger, has been used by herbalists to warm the body since ancient times. The Indonesians use it for flavouring, improving the appetite, aiding digestion and helping with rheumatic pain. Pickled ginger has long been used to prevent motion sickness and is now recommended for morning sickness in Western books on natural healing. Ginger teas are becoming increasingly popular for nausea.

Indonesians believe its juice works well for colic, coughs and catarrh. The pounded rhizome is also good for itching, grazes and deep wounds, and one of its prime functions in Indonesia is warming the body. When combined with salt, a smaller variety of ginger root (*surti; Zingiber officinale* var. *rubrum*) is an important antidote for snake bites.

Common ginger appears in formulæ for Galian Langsing, a slimming jamu for men and women; Galian Singset, to tighten and firm the body; Galian Gadis, for teenage health; Sehat Wanita, to give women energy and good health; Sehat Lelaki, which does the same for men; Galian Bersalin for post-natal care; Hamil Tua, for problems in late pregnancy, and Sawan for itchiness and stomach upsets in babies. Finally, common ginger is used in tonics and medicines for stimulating the appetite.

Turmeric (*Curcuma domestica*)

Turmeric has travelled way beyond the kitchen. The rhizome's botanical name, *Curcuma domestica*, comes from the Arabic *kurkum*, but Indonesians call it *kunyit* or *kunir* (*kunyit* in Indonesian; *kunir* in Javanese), meaning yellow. Turmeric has added flavour and colour to Asian cooking for thousands of years. It provides the yellow in curries and is used to colour dishes for ritual celebrations, such as the Indonesian rice cone known as a *tumpeng*.

Colour is the key to turmeric's history. Yellow has long been considered sacred in the East because it symbolizes the sun, the source of light, energy and growth. Thus, it is associated with royalty throughout Asia. In some cases turmeric is used as a substitute for saffron. It is widely believed that turmeric offers protection against evil spirits, which accounts for its prominence in Hindu culture and at weddings and circumcision ceremonies in Indonesia. Buddhist monks use turmeric to dye their robes and in the 13th century, turmeric caught the attention of the inveterate explorer, Marco Polo, who noticed it growing in southern China. Despite its healing ability, turmeric has more frequently been used as a dye and food flavouring.

The association of turmeric with the yellow of royalty is evident in the fabric, food and beauty treatments of the Central Javanese palaces. Even today, court ladies are still massaged with *lulur* paste coloured with turmeric to give their skin the preferred golden glow. (It is not, however, recommended for

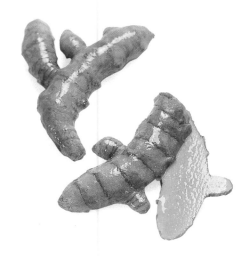

Above:
With a wealth of history behind it, deep-yellow turmeric is used for cosmetic and medicinal purposes throughout the archipelago.

Caucasian skins.) In Central Java, the paste is often coloured with another little-known member of the ginger family, *temu giring* (*Curcuma heyneana*), or a mixture of the two gingers. It is significant that manufacturer, Sari Ayu, makes as many as 16 jamu containing turmeric for women. These formulæ cover almost every requirement from radiant complexion, slimming, rejuvenation, post-natal and hair treatments, to poultices and compresses that cleanse and deodorize. Turmeric also goes into Jamu Asih Kinasih, the love potion that is said to bring a whole new meaning to the word love-making.

Asian healers' faith in the curative powers of turmeric has been endorsed by modern science. Turmeric has anti-bacterial, anti-fungal and anti-viral properties; it also contains an active chemical called curcumin, which can reduce inflammation by up to 50 per cent. In some instances, it even successfully out-performs steroids. Osteoarthritic patients are often prescribed a formula based on turmeric, and it is also taken for rheumatism. As a bonus, science has proven that curcumin has anti-mutagenic properties and can help protect living cells from substances that cause cancer. As with certain vitamins, curcumin apparently functions like an antioxidant.

Traditional thinking says turmeric is the answer to liver problems and jaundice. Again, modern scientists agree, as turmeric increases the flow of bile that causes the gall bladder to contract and helps prevent the formation of gallstones. Secondly, extra bile means fat in the intestine is digested more efficiently, thus turmeric has a hand in reducing cholesterol and cleaning the blood. This double action explains why it is often found in herbal slimming pills in the West.

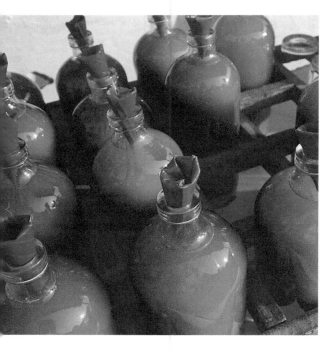

Above:
*Bottled Kunir Asem,
a typical product sold
by Indonesian men.
Generally men choose
to sell jamu that does
not deal with sexual or
female complaints, to
avoid embarrassment.*

Even without the benefit of scientific evidence, Indonesians have always believed in turmeric. This is obvious from the millions of people who swallow a glass of the turmeric-rich Jamu Kunir Asem on a daily basis, thus lining the system with a mild, antiseptic wash. This habit is important in a country where food is often cooked in the morning, then covered and left out all day in the heat, a practice that can lead to stomach infections. Indonesians see turmeric primarily as a disinfectant, but a secondary use is to combat stomach ache and diarrhoea.

Turmeric is found in practically every jamu, since Indonesians rightly believe that it is anti-inflammatory and a painkiller that both cleanses the blood and improves circulation. Its other attributes include reducing bleeding, and healing wounds, itchiness, ulcers and abscesses. Burnt and inhaled, it relieves a stuffy nose and plays a role in treating asthma, angina, hypertension and fever. Combined with other ingredients, turmeric is a remedy for ailments as diverse as sore, cracked skin, post-natal problems, eczema, stomach abscesses, sores and dysentery.

We learn from the great Dutch botanist Rumphius (who was in fact German-born Georg Everard Rumpf, 1628–1702) that turmeric had another function: "…these same flowers are also of use against Fire-Piss or Gonorrhey, in both Men and Women." His recommendation? Mix seven unopened flower buds with young coconut and the problem disappears.

Turmeric is known by 80 different names in Indonesia's thousands of villages, which gives some measure of its importance. The plant likes fertile, well-aerated soil and grows more or less anywhere below 600 metres (1,200 feet), so it is widely available. Its smell is at once fresh and musky, the taste is pungent with a hint of ginger and a touch of orange. The darker the rhizome, the better the quality; it also needs to grow for a year before it can be used in medicine.

Today's scientists have compared the rhizome's action to that of modern aspirin although its list of applications seems more impressive. Recently two Indian doctors living in the United States added a new twist to the turmeric tale. In 1995, they were granted a patent on the healing effects of turmeric powder. The move caused immediate uproar in India, where turmeric and its healing powers are regarded as common property. The row escalated into a major legal battle, which the doctors lost. Thus, the medicinal value of turmeric was thrust into the limelight in the West.

Resurrection lily (*kencur*; *Kaempferia galanga*)

Largely unknown outside Asia, this rhizome played a part in European medieval herbalism and is still important in Indonesian cuisine. Nothing can replace its sharp, slightly camphor-like taste in soups, sauces, curries and stews. Malays call this root *chekur*. The rhizome is sometimes wrongly identified by Western cookery writers, most of whom have never seen it fresh, as zedoary (*Curcuma zedoaria*) or lesser galangal (*Alpinia officinarum*). To avoid any possible confusion, this book uses the Indonesian name throughout.

Kencur root is always used in warming remedies, and is recommended for over 20 illnesses—including chills in elephants! Because *kencur* warms the body, thus causing it to perspire, it is effectively used for poultice and compress pastes,

63

and for treating fever, muscular rheumatism, abdominal pain, stomach ache and swelling. For instance, a well-proven cure for swelling is massaging the affected area with ground *kencur*, lemon grass and salt. In every Javanese household, the antidote to coughs and colds is a drink of pressed *kencur* juice, while rheumatism, sore muscles and joints are treated with Jamu Beras Kencur (a mixture of *kencur*, rice, sugar, salt and tamarind). This jamu is known to increase appetite, so is not recommended for dieters.

The credibility of *kencur* is reinforced by its regular medicinal application in other cultures. For centuries, the Chinese used *kencur* for stomach upsets and duodenal ulcers, and it featured prominently in ancient Egyptian medicine. In the Philippines, it is used for colds and headaches. Thais use *kencur* in the kitchen and also for headaches, while sailors who transported *kencur* to Europe for culinary purposes, as medicine or catarrh-relieving snuff, quickly discovered it made an excellent antidote to sea sickness.

In recent experiments on breathing difficulties, menthol, camphor and *kencur* were mixed, one at a time, with oil and balsam. The *kencur* mix turned out to be the most successful. When small quantities were used, an improvement was seen in 20 minutes, but when the *kencur* content was increased to 30 per cent, the same level of improvement was obvious within five minutes.

Kencur is also an ingredient in health and beauty preparations formulated to resolve hormonal problems. If the body is unbalanced or needs a general tonic, the answer might lie in Jamu Awet Ayu, a rejuvenating jamu. Most of these beauty

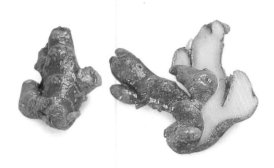

Above:
Used throughout Asia for its healing qualities, kencur *was part of the European healing arsenal during medieval times, but subsequently disappeared, as no further text references to the rhizome were found after medieval times.*

formulæ read like a ginger family reunion and nearly always include the *kencur* rhizome.

Kencur is officially considered the seventh most popular jamu ingredient. Consequently, scientists are searching for the best ways to cultivate it. They know the rhizome has a preference for loose, crumbly, sandy soil, a particular penchant for peaty, woody, mossy places and will flourish up to 900 metres (2,700 feet). Active projects centre on how to protect it from insects and disease, as well as choosing the right nutrients, fertilisers and conditions to produce a perfect rhizome. Scientists are currently evaluating *kencur* as an insecticide and preliminary reports indicate it could help eradicate Asia's dangerous Aedes mosquito larvae responsible for dengue fever.

Greater galangal (*laos* or *lengkuas*; *Languas galanga*)

The use of greater galangal (commonly referred to as galangal in English) in healing practice can be traced back to the 6th and 7th centuries, when it was prescribed by physicians in countries as far apart as India, Arabia and Greece. The Arabs even believed galangal was an aphrodisiac. Three hundred years later, records show galangal was added to medicine by the Chinese and according to scientist Isaac Henry Burkill, by AD 1200 they were exporting it to Palembang in Sumatra. Marco Polo tells us that the Javanese grew and supplied galangal to the spice traders in the 13th century.

Twelve kinds of galangal are widely used in Indonesian medicine, but the most popular variety is *Languas galanga*, used in jamu for indigestion, stomach aches, diarrhoea and flatulence. Its active compound is cineol, a proven antiseptic.

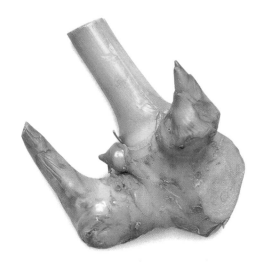

Below:
Lengkuas or galangal is a native of Java and the Malay Peninsula and is widely used for medicinal and culinary purposes in Southeast Asia.

Specializing in Tempuyung

Bapak Partono lives on the outskirts of Yogyakarta where he runs a business dedicated to growing *tempuyung* (*Sonchus arvensis*) or, as it is dubbed locally, kidney stone leaves. Bapak Partono discovered, on analysis, that his garden soil was particularly rich in calcium oxalat, a calcium known for its healing properties. The theory is that the calcium in the *tempuyung* leaves can wipe out the calcium build-up in the kidneys. He likened it to washing salt-water fish in saline water to remove the excess salt.

His small business involves growing, drying, sorting and selecting suitable leaves for jamu. After an initial drying in a warm cupboard at temperatures of 40-60°C, the leaves are trussed up on bamboo racks and dried in the air or, in some cases, dried over a fire in an enamel, not metal, pot as they cannot come into contact with iron.

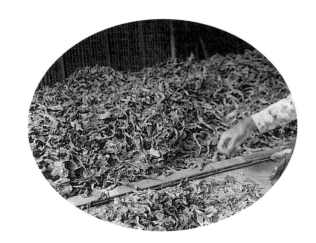

"We don't get any problems with fungus," explains Bapak Partono, "because the leaves are not dried directly by fire or under the sun." Rejected leaves are thrown out, not, as in the case of some factories, recycled with chemical additives.

"I run a traditional business and refuse to have synthetic materials tangled up in the production process," he says. Generally, his success rate is high and patients report a marked improvement after the first month of taking *tempuyung*. With the assistance of Professor Dr Ismadi (the Head of Biochemistry at Gadjah Mada University in Yogyakarta), Bapak Partono works hard to ensure on-going quality control and is also looking at ways of improving his growing methods.

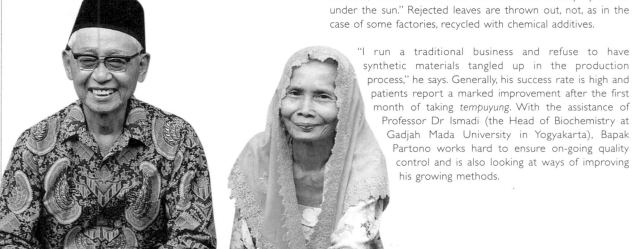

Kudu Laos is a typical jamu formula based on galangal. The recipe is a good example of how jamu ingredients interact to achieve an effective result. It cures indigestion, wind and loss of appetite. Among other ingredients, this jamu combines the curing properties of galangal with garlic—antiseptic, anti-bacteria and anti-inflammatory—and because both ingredients are full of natural vitamins and minerals, the potion also boosts overall health. Kudu Laos also includes *mengkudu* (Indian mulberry; *Morinda citrifolia*), a laxative that is also especially recommended for liver complaints; white pepper for its warming effect; young tamarind, which contains vitamin B, for wind and diarrhoea; and white sugar, Javanese brown sugar and salt. All these ingredients are selected to enhance one another's chemical action.

Writing on the Moluccas at the end of the 17th century, the knowledgeable Dr Rumphius informs us galangal was pounded with leaves and pepper as a cure for severe scurf and other skin problems, and was prescribed for herpes sufferers as a last and drastic resort. It is also known that innocuous ingredients like galangal were often included in deadly poisons, but we do not know any logical reason for this.

As a culinary flavouring, galangal appears in many Indonesian dishes such as *rendang* and curry, or in fish and chicken recipes. It is a cornerstone in South Sulawesi's hearty beef stews for which the province is famous. One advantage of galangal is its ability to grow almost anywhere, although it thrives in a dry, sunny spot. For culinary use, the rhizome is dug up two-and-a-half to three months after planting; left in the ground any longer, it becomes unpleasantly fibrous. Greater galangal grows

---

Red Rice makes a Comeback

Decades ago, millions of young Indonesians were brought up on *beras merah* or red rice, as it was a cheaper alternative to the so-called white rice. As with all rice that is not polished, its husk is particularly rich in vitamin B1 and is useful in treating certain complaints. Red rice is particularly effective in treating upset and bloated stomachs. The medicinal qualities are brought out by roasting (note: not frying) two dessert spoons of red rice and then steeping this in a glass of boiling water. When the water has turned a rich shade of red, the liquid is ready to drink.

to a height of around two metres (six feet) and its rhizome turns from pale pinkish purple when young, to orangey red when mature. It has a fresh smell and tastes of ginger and pepper, with a hint of sour lemon.

Temu lawak (or temu besar; Curcuma xanthorrhiza)

This useful rhizome has no common English name, the nearest translation of its Javanese name being old rhizome, from *temu* (rhizome) and *lawak* (old). However, the other Indonesian name, *temu besar* meaning big rhizome, is an accurate description. Like turmeric and galangal, its prime function is to stimulate digestion and release bile from the gall bladder. It is also popular for a range of ailments from diarrhoea and constipation, to fever, muscle spasms and skin complaints; it increases the flow of milk during breastfeeding and improves blood circulation.

The deep yellow colour of *temu lawak* may explain why it is often prescribed for jaundice and liver complaints, as per the doctrine of signatures theory mentioned earlier. It is also blessed with a pungent smell and bitter taste. Like any other jamu remedy, *temu lawak*'s properties change depending on what goes into the mixture. For example, for years Indonesians have cured itchy skin by mixing desiccated sap from the stem of a mousedeer's eye plant (*mata pelandok*; *Ardisia elliptica*) with coconut oil and *temu lawak*.

Charles Ong, President Director of Nyonya Meneer, is so convinced of its efficacy he was prepared to publicly support clinical trial evidence that showed a combination of turmeric and *temu lawak* relieved the symptoms of rheumatism. Along

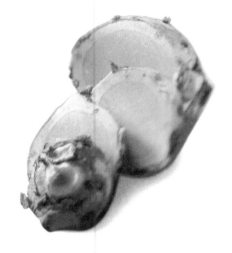

Above:
Temu lawak *was advocated by Mrs Kloppenburg who used it in over 50 of her herbal remedies.*

with *sidowayah* (grandchild's arrival; *Woodfordia fruticosa*), *kunci pepet* (white turmeric; *Kaempferia rotunda*) (a cooling turmeric containing cineol) and Javanese long pepper (*cabe jawa*; *Piper retrofractum*), *temu lawak* is put into Sari Ayu's Perawatan Wanita (Ladies Care Tablets) to give busy women a lift by improving the blood and restoring muscle tone.

Its popularity is borne out by Mrs Kloppenburg-Versteegh (see page 16), who included *temu lawak* in no less than 51 recipes in her book of herbal remedies, eight of which are for liver complaints. She also exhorts anyone with abdominal problems to take it neat, despite another school of thought that says this root should always be mixed with at least five other ingredients.

This ginger's therapeutic value was also endorsed by a French traveller named LeClerc, who wrote a learned thesis on it during the 19th century. Tales of the rhizome's success in liver and gallstone treatments led to large quantities being exported to Holland in the 1800s, where they were made into infusions and drunk two or three times a day. In the 1980s, it appeared on the Dutch list of pharmaceutical specialities and the Netherlands Drug Bulletin affirmed *temu lawak*'s extensive use for gall bladder complaints.

In Holland, it is sold fresh, powdered or in tablet form. The root also plays a part in cosmetics, where full use is made of its medicinal properties in face and body care preparations. For instance, it is an ingredient in Galian Kempes Perut, which slims by removing fats, cleansing the blood and eliminating waste. It is also found in Galian Singset, guaranteed to make the body firm and tight, internally and externally, by removing liquids rather than fats. It is an even-tempered plant that grows in most places between one to 500 metres (three feet to 1,500 feet). Whilst *temu lawak* is cultivated in Java, it can still be found growing wild in the teak forests elsewhere in the Indonesian archipelago.

Lempuyang (*lempuyang pahit; Zingiber amaricans* and *lempuyang wangi; Zingiber aromaticum*)
The last of the high profile gingers is *lempuyang*, also without a common English name though it is sometimes called wild or bitter ginger. The principle task of this plant is to warm the body and increase muscle flexibility. It is known for its strong flavour and extremely biting, bitter taste. This makes it a popular appetiser seasoning, because it activates taste buds. Consequently, juice from *lempuyang* roots is often prescribed as medicine to stimulate the appetite after illness.

Draughts are prescribed for stomach pains accompanied by cramps in the legs. *Lempuyang* is applied externally to treat fever and numbness in the feet. The rhizome's irritants draw blood to a certain part of the body by over-stimulating blood vessels and nerves. This causes the skin to redden, thus increasing the blood flow and cleansing the tissues of toxins.

The root is frequently used to heal infections after childbirth and it is an effective tonic. Crushed *lempuyang* mixed with coconut oil and ash becomes a paste that is smeared over hard swellings to reduce the inflammation. Change the ingredients to *lempuyang*, roasted red onions and liquorice strained through a cloth and it becomes a cure for whooping cough—another example of jamu's versatility.

Lempuyang is an active ingredient in Jamu Pria Awet Muda (Forever Young jamu). Until recently, this formula was the exclusive property of Javanese royalty and one of the secrets of their excellent health, youthful looks and long life. *Temu lawak* is put into the male version that keeps men fit, virile and energetic whatever their age. Ladies of the court have their own variety called Wanita Awet Muda, but this formula is based on ginger and *kayu pahit* (translated as bitter bark), a green shrub (*Strychnos ligustrina*).

A Cornucopia of Spices
Spices used in jamu include cinnamon, nutmeg, mace, cloves, fennel, black and white pepper, cardamom, coriander, cumin and caraway seeds, together with herbs such as basil, dried tamarind fruit and brown or white sugar. With the availability of over 1,000 medicinal plants, the range of combinations is said to cure most maladies. Common additions to these plants include papaya, betel leaves, chilli peppers, orange or pomegranate skins and bastard cedar, or any of the 900 or so on the WHO list. Jamu Kunir Asem illustrates how different mixes effect different cures. Sold as a healthy tonic, it is transformed into a slimming recipe when betel leaf is added.

What do these spices contribute? Cinnamon (*Cinnamomum zeylanicum*) brings flavour and freshness to the drink, while nutmeg (*Myristica fragrans*) adds taste and has a calming effect because it is a narcotic medicinal compound. Nutmeg helps wind, indigestion and stomach problems, but it can be highly toxic in very large doses owing to the chemical myristicin, which can cause convulsions and in some cases, abortion.

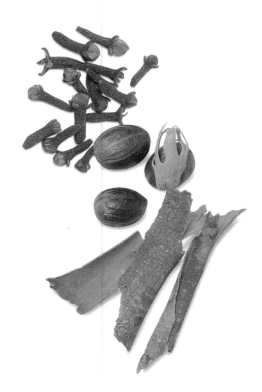

Nutmeg and cloves (*Syzgium aromatica*) both stop diarrhoea, while the latter is prescribed for stomach pain, nausea or vomiting. Fennel has a similar action on the stomach and bowels; it regulates urine flow and brings down fevers as well.

Pepper (*Piper* sp.) concentrates on warming, but also destroys parasites and removes gas. White pepper (which is simply the ripe peppercorn with the wrinkled black skin removed) works as a diuretic and a contraceptive, while its leaves go into remedies for leprosy and eczema. Black pepper's specialities are removing phlegm, purifying the blood and treating rheumatism. Cardamom (*Elettaria cardamomum*), coriander (*Coriandrum sativum*), and cumin (*Cuminum cyminum*) are a valuable trio. Cardamom takes care of coughs, rheumatism, itchy skin and fever. Coriander clears up indigestion and nausea. Black cumin is warming and good for stomach ache, while the white variety increases metabolic activity and helps stomach pain.

Curative Poisons

Pharmacists, botanists and doctors all admit there is a thin line between curing and poisoning. The decisive factor in prescribing jamu is the size of the dose and, where necessary, the addition of a neutralizing plant to counteract toxicity. Many jamu ingredients appear on the WHO Priority List of the most used medicinal plants, yet they are toxic. Tamarind (*Tamarindus indica*), for example, is accorded this 'privilege'. Although the entire plant is poisonous, its medicinal use is widespread. The young leaves are applied externally for healing skin diseases, ulcers and rheumatism and are a good source of vitamin B, while tamarind pulp (frequently used in cooking) is cooling, and

Above:
Cloves, nutmeg and cinnamon, three spices that contributed to the famous Spice Routes in the 19th century.

acts as a gentle laxative. The stronger pulp of old fruits, known as *asem kawak*, is recommended for those who seek an abortion. Similarly, the sap of the cashew nut tree (*Anacardium occidentale*) is poisonous, although the nuts themselves are edible. Mixed with powdered lime, the leaves are made into a poultice for skin diseases and burns. The roots are a laxative and the bark makes an effective gargle. However, the oily juice of the fruit skin, prescribed for warts and skin ulcers, can produce a sharp reaction because it contains a toxic tannin called cardol, and anacardic acid. Furthermore, the pounded fruit is a homeopathic cure for psychological problems like loss of memory, overwork and poor sexual performance.

The leaves, roots and seeds of *kecubung* (horn of plenty; *Datura metal*) are highly toxic. Nonetheless, its roots are used in remedies for cholera, asthma and toothache, while the leaves relieve lower back pain, swelling and rheumatism. In modern medicinal application, *Datura metal* is important because it can reduce spasms by blocking the action of part of the nervous system. Thieves often prepare a narcotic powder from the seeds to spray over their intended victims putting them into a deep sleep, but this crime can unwittingly become murder if the dosage is too strong.

The deceptively pretty pink flowers of the Madagascar periwinkle (*Catharanthus roseus*) are both a useful healer and a lethal poison. Yet the plant is revered as a miracle cure for certain forms of cancer. Another questionable plant is the green, leafy physic nut (*Jatropha curcas*): Although the psychic nut is on the WHO Priority List, its seeds contain two poisons that can burn the throat and damage the intestines. It is often

Below:
Coriander is highly nutritious; rich in calcium, phosphorus and vitamin C, it is curiously a native of southern Europe.

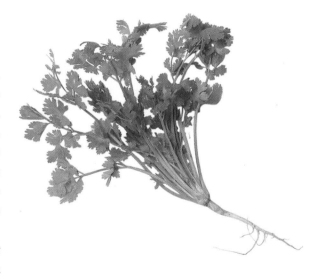

taken for edema, dropsy, or as a liniment for rheumatism, skin diseases and hair growth, but accidental cases of poisoning are still common in Asia.

The four o'clock flower (*Mirabilis jalapa*), so called because it opens in the late afternoon, has poisonous roots and seeds. Yet the root is taken for chronic constipation, while its seeds are a mild laxative and, when crushed into a fine powder, are used to make face powder. The humble pineapple (*Ananas* sp.) and lovely yellow allamanda flowers (*Allamanda* sp.) (great for fevers and diarrhoea) often cause contact dermatitis. Used correctly, these 'dangerous plants' become efficient healers. But, as in Western medicine, the effectiveness of a treatment really all depends on the skill of the practitioner.

Dwindling Resources
The greatest problem facing today's traditional medicine makers is disappearing raw materials. Most ingredients are found in the wild, and over-exploitation of these natural resources has meant some medicinal plants have become endangered. In many cases we have no Western names for these valuable products. At this moment in time, there are 15 plants vital for many jamu approaching extinction. Some of these plants may be irreplaceable, and while rainforests continue to shrink, others are lost before their healing powers are even discovered.

Pulosari (*Alyxia stellata*), a white bark found in almost every Javanese jamu, is under threat. It is often present to mask the taste and smell of other raw materials but is particularly well known as a remedy for coughs, fever, urinary problems and gonorrhoea. The same danger applies to *sintok* (*Cinnamomum sintoc*), a reddish-brown bark prescribed for many illnesses, including diarrhoea, insect bites and syphilis.

Temu mangga (*Curcuma mangga*) is a favourite culinary seasoning. It doubles up as a remedy for stomach problems and fever, but is almost impossible to buy in local markets nowadays. *Masoyi* (*Cryptocarya massoy*), a popular perfume for incense and also widely used for cramps during pregnancy, is fast disappearing as well. *Jenitri* (*Elaeocarpus ganitrus*) is the Java laurel tree; its gall is used for treating white vaginal discharge and pus in the womb, and the tree is becoming scarce.

One of the stalwarts of slimming jamu, the bastard cedar (*Guazuma ulmifolia*; *jati belanda*), is now in danger. The same is true of *kayu rapet* (*Parameria laevigata*), the bark used in recipes to keep a woman's body and complexion in beautiful condition. Its prime function is to dry and tighten the vagina. It is a favourite product of many Indonesian women who will, however, feign embarrassment at the mention of the name and suggest that this jamu is "only for bad girls".

Burahol (*Stelechocarpus burahol*), whose fruit removes smell from the urine, is also part of this sorry tale, as is *purwoceng* (*Pimpinella alpina*), which (as its name suggests) grows high up in the mountains. It is considered a wonderful aphrodisiac and impotency cure, and goes into countless remedies. *Kikoneng* (*Arcangelisia flava*) has, in its stem, chemical components useful for treating jaundice, mouth ulcers and smallpox, while the seeds are an antidote for poisoning. Its numbers are also decreasing.

Well-known names on the endangered species list are the perfumes, sandalwood (*Santalum album*) and musk mallow (*Abelmoschus moschatus*; *gandapura* or fragrance of the palace).

Apart from adding their famous scents to jamu cosmetics, they soften skin, are used in face powders and can effectively treat rheumatics or wind.

An unusual member of the group is *kayu angin* (*Usnea thallus*), whose Indonesian name means 'windy wood'. This pale grey lichen hangs from trees in high, moist, windy places, and is an astringent and anti-spasmodic that helps intestinal problems and bowel complaints. People burned *kayu angin* in the house, believing the lichen could combat evil spirits and wind-borne disease in the same way it filtered wind when hanging down from the branches of trees.

Kayu ular (*Strychnos lucida*) and *sidowayah* (*Woodfordia fruticosa*) are two essentials for tonics, constipation and bowel remedies. Both are used in medium to large amounts, and because of their rarity, are becoming very expensive.

As it is impossible to find substitutes for many of these plants and trees, botanists would like to see their natural habitats designated as conservation areas and protected by government regulation. Another option is to follow a selective picking system. One such example is a scheme already operating on the Dieng Plateau in Central Java, where people living in the vicinity are allowed only to pick shoots from the top of the *purwoceng* plant, leaving the rest of the plant alone to encourage its recovery and regrowth.

To handle what is fast becoming an emergency, it makes sense to enlist the aid of professionals at the botanical and medicinal plant gardens who have the expertise to store seeds, pollen or tissue cultures. If special plantations are set up, the outlook is promising. If not, the loss of vitally important plants is inevitable. Geography has made Indonesia custodian of approximately 10 per cent of the world's plants. This quirk of nature means that the country is under enormous pressure from scientific communities worldwide to take better care of her natural heritage. The dilemma its leaders now face is how to simultaneously preserve this legacy for the future and continue reaping its benefits, without destroying the resources they are trying to preserve.

Why We Still Need Plants
With ample supplies of synthetic drugs nowadays, do we really need nature's help anymore? Surprisingly, nearly 40 per cent of modern medicines is derived from plants, so the answer is clear. Also, in the past decade, the unpleasant side effects that accompany certain drugs have encouraged some Westerners to return to natural therapies. Many Indonesians who have tasted Western medicine are also returning to old-fashioned, natural remedies. Consequently, demand for medicinal herbs has risen.

Between 1989 and 1993, overall jamu production rose by almost 159 per cent, while total jamu sales shot up by a healthy 63 per cent. Exports showed a less impressive increase of 32 per cent, only because by the time the home market had taken its pick, there was not much left to export. Nyonya Meneer's factory more than doubled its output during this time, but this was still not enough to meet demand. Since that period, it has been difficult to obtain statistics, but jamu sales seem to have stabilized: with recent economic troubles at home, people have less money to spend on Western medicines, and often revert to traditional formulae.

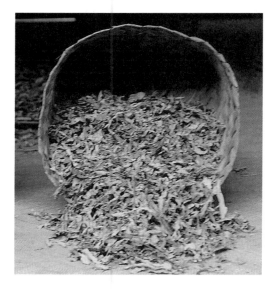

Above:
Tempuyung or kidney stone leaves, ready for processing. Tempuyung is rich in calcium oxalat and is used in jamu that rids the kidneys of calcium build-up.

To meet the challenge, entrepreneurs are racing to modernize factories and set up new plantations. A recent Ministry of Health survey on the medicinal herb industry estimated it would soon need 8,000 tonnes of herbs a year to meet the demand for herbal medicine. But, even Indonesia's fertile land will not make plants and trees shoot up overnight, and the country's medicinal plant experts are currently looking at the production problem, trying to determine ideal growing conditions and to improve efficiency. Handled correctly, plants often respond positively and this might prove the answer to yet another hurdle in the expansion of the industry.

Given the right conditions, what can go wrong? Quite a lot, apparently. Active ingredients are only present at certain stages in a plant's growth cycle. At times the ingredients can be too strong or too weak. Roots and leaves also vary in taste depending on whether the rhizome is cultivated, or grown in the wild. Temperature, altitude and soil conditions are all very important factors in plant growth, and some jamu simply need plants or herbs that are grown in certain conditions if they are to be effective.

Take *kencur*. Make Jamu Beras Kencur with *kencur* from Central Java and it tastes delicious. Buy *kencur* around Jakarta, where soil is normally red rather than black and it can taste tart. On the other hand, try *kencur* from a market on Batam Island near Singapore, and you will find it so small, young and bitter that you will never want to repeat the experience again. Anyone who has tried removing skin from these tiny and knobbly, *kencur* rhizomes will confirm the job has nervous breakdown potential.

The Economic and the Botanic Gardens

The colonial Dutch were quick to realize there was money to be made if they could standardize and improve the quality of Indonesia's natural resources. In the early 1800s, they established two research centres at Bogor, in the hills south of Jakarta, where climate, altitude and soil provided perfect growing conditions.

These twin pillars, the Economic and the Botanical Gardens had one purpose: to collect, cultivate and conduct scientific research into plants and crops. They specialized in different areas of research but shared their results, a strategy that allowed rapid progress. The Economic Garden introduced new plants, cultivated them, improved the strain and passed specimens to farmers for testing. The Garden's commercial bias meant it concentrated on plants already in demand, such as quinine. In the 1930s, quinine was the only known cure for malaria and Indonesia supplied 80 per cent of the world's requirement.

The Economic Garden also worked on herbs and spices with commercial potential. It researched plants like *kumis kucing* (cat's whiskers; *Orthosiphon aristatus*), *temu lawak* (*Curcuma xanthorrhiza*) and *akar tuba* (*Derris elliptica*; a climber used as fish poison and, at one time, the toxic component for insecticides). They cultivated patchouli, lemon grass, vetiver, sandalwood and *kenanga* (ylang-ylang; *Canangium odoratum*) for use in perfume and beauty preparations. Their range of spices focused on black pepper, cinnamon, cloves, cubeb pepper, ginger, cardamom and vanilla—all names that were already sought after in Europe's kitchens. The Botanical Garden was equally productive. It started from nothing in 1817, but

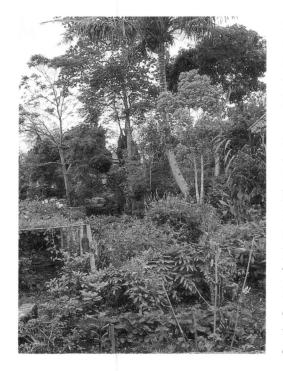

50 years later boasted over 10,000 different species. By 1876, the Garden was forced to acquire new land for expansion and experimental work. The momentum continued, and a year later, the Director founded Indonesia's first Agricultural School, the Plant and Veterinary Institute.

These developments laid the foundations for Bogor's internationally acclaimed botanical and agricultural research centres. Facilities now include a Herbarium and Ballitro, an institute for the study of medicinal plants. Both are staffed by highly qualified scientists who are gradually proving that Indonesian medicinal plants can make a major contribution to world health. There are also experimental gardens in Lembang, West Java, and the mountaintop village of Tawangmangu outside Solo. As one scientist said: "The Indonesian way of life has changed and we are in serious danger of losing our rarest plants and trees. Unless we act now, valuable sources of medicine could disappear before we have even discovered them."

Curative Remedies or Culinary Concoctions?
Roughly half the ingredients in any Indonesian dish are also used for traditional medicine cures. As the well-known Australian herbalist, Dorothy Hall, asked: "When does a plant cease being a food and become a medicine? This question has bugged me for years because I can't answer it. What is the difference, say, between celery eaten as a vegetable and celery extract prescribed by a herbalist as a medicine?"

John Naisbitt, author of *Megatrends Asia* and co-author of *Megatrends 2000*, two books that focus on economic forecasts in

Above:
The attractive Experimental Garden at Tawangmangu. In September and October, when the medicinal plants are in bloom, the gardens are at their best.

the Asian region, believes "some of the impetus to accept food as medicine comes from a new emphasis on natural healthful foods, as well as influences from Far Eastern cultures and new scientific discoveries". Adding curing herbs to food is probably less effective than drinking the same roots and leaves in jamu, because quantities are smaller and hence less concentrated. Even assuming jamu's deliberate chemical reaction is missing in a dish, the cumulative, advantageous effect of eating these healthy herbs and spices on a daily basis cannot be ignored. They are the body's regular top-up of essential vitamins and minerals, which might otherwise be lacking in the diet.

In the tropics, dishes vary with the season. The dry season sees families eating more sour foods like cooling vegetables, sour sugar and saffron. The rainy season encourages Indonesians to take warming drinks such as ginger, and to cook with large amounts of coconut.

Looking at some of the common foods in Indonesia, we see that starfruit reduces blood pressure, while its cooling effect works wonders for scurvy and whooping cough. The leaves are a cure for rheumatism. Boiled in water, they are a remedy for fever or diabetes and possess certain antibiotic properties. The juice of the thin-skinned lime (*Citrus aurantifolia*) when mixed with *daun sirih* (betel leaves), salt and hot water is effective in the treatment of itchy rashes. After two or three applications, the rash usually disappears.

As already discussed, turmeric has antiseptic powers, and capsaicin, the compound that gives the bite to chillies, aids respiration. Candlenuts, which are added to vegetable dishes and soups, gently clean out the system. Meanwhile scientific

Below:
Candlenuts, native to Malaysia and Indonesia, have purgative qualities.

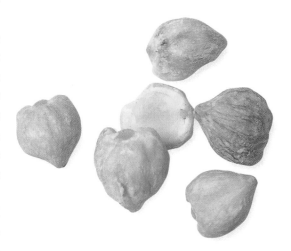

tests have revealed that mango, another Indonesian favourite, contains two compounds to prevent the herpes virus duplicating itself, thus effectively killing it off.

People of the archipelago have learned what healthy ingredients are over centuries. They thrived on a diet of fresh leaves and fruits that contained healthy enzymes. When they were sick, a quick stroll around the neighbourhood to pick up a few medicinal barks and plants was the equivalent of dropping in at the local pharmacy. Experience taught them what to look for, and their fertile plains or rich rain forests, ensured an abundant supply. Food provided life's essentials in terms of vitamins, minerals, carbohydrates and proteins. As in many other Asian countries, Indonesians were aware of how food could also be used as medicine.

These healthy eating habits comprise a well-balanced macro diet. Based on rice, vegetables, nuts, pulses and fresh fruit, the intake is supplemented by soya beans and small portions of fish or meat. The final touch is the vast range of spices which seasons main dishes and appears in a variety of hot sambal sauces such as chilli, shallot, yam bean, mango and dried shrimp paste. Combining these ingredients helps ward off all sorts of diseases including cancer, high blood pressure, cholesterol and heart problems.

Moving With the Times
Nowadays, 'progress' is slowly eroding traditional eating patterns. Hamburgers, milk, cheese and yoghurt have long made their debut in Indonesia and show no sign of departing. Not surprisingly, government statistics indicate cancer and hyper-

tension have increased dramatically, while heart disease is now the number one killer in Indonesia's larger cities. The good news is that traditional foods are still easily available. One of the tourist attractions of Indonesia is the sight of mobile food sellers announcing their home-cooked fare day and night; markets are thriving: these are busy places where you can always get a quick but delicious meal at a food stall.

At one time, cooks were also experts on medicinal foods. Every Javanese family had its *botekan*, a storage box for around 15 kinds of herbs and spices. Most of its contents had a dual purpose, because they went into both the cooking pot and the herbal medicine concoction. Today, the skill has largely disappeared as women juggle their time between family and work. They buy from a favourite street seller or rustle up something quick and tasty. Recipes have survived but few people know if, or what, they can cure.

Having served as a distillation point for different cultures, Indonesia has been influenced by the diets and ancient medical systems of four different cultures, namely Indian, European, Arab and Chinese. All support, to varying degrees, the theory that proper nutrition is the key to good health. Food, medicine and power of the mind have long been seen as a single entity.

The Kitchen Apothecary

Food does not count as jamu, though this depends, of course, on how you define jamu and how you prepare it. However, food does count as traditional medicine. Many of the basic ingredients in the Indonesian kitchen are rhizomes, herbs and spices. Gingers include common ginger, turmeric, Chinese keys and

Below:
A botekan, *or herbal storage chest.*

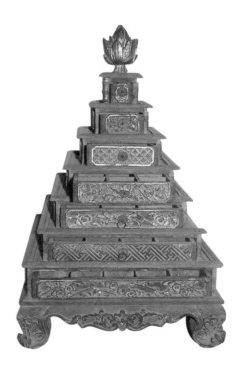

83

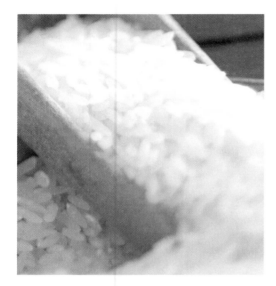

Above:
Rice—the staple food in Indonesia is equally useful in making jamu and many of the beauty preparations of yester-year as well as modern skincare products.

kencur. The dried spices include black and white pepper, coriander, nutmeg, cumin and cloves. In addition, Indonesian cooks use tamarind, candlenuts, brown sugar, *salam* leaves (similar in appearance although not in flavour to bay leaves), lemon grass, kaffir limes, chilli, red onions, garlic and dried shrimp paste.

To explain this concept, examples of food that double as medicine are included below. The ingredients are typically Indonesian, found on every table, grown in the villages, or bought in local markets.

Rice (Oryza sativa)

No Indonesian meal would be complete without rice, and the popular tonic, Jamu Beras Kencur, depends on it. Visitors travelling through parts of Indonesia are impressed by the endless terraces of immaculately cultivated paddy fields, which represent a livelihood to the people they feed. Consequently, rice features prominently in numerous ceremonies and celebrations in Indonesia. Births, deaths, marriages, a new venture, boat or house—all receive their fair share of rice in some shape or form. The *tumpeng* or yellow rice cone coloured with turmeric takes pride of place on most of these occasions.

As food, rice adds protein, fat, carbohydrate and ash to the diet. Beriberi, which causes inflammation of the nerves and results from a deficiency of vitamin B, is often treated with rice polishings because they are rich in this vitamin. Western research has recently announced that rice starch protects against cancer. The starch can also be scented and used to make a cooling face powder. Powdered rice, consisting mainly of rice starch or *bedak*, the base for Indonesian cosmetics, is coloured and prescribed as a magic cure for sickness. The shade changes with the time of day: "white in the morning, red at midday and black at sundown".

At one time, combining rice starch with pepper was a remedy for 'gouty twinges' in the hands and feet, as noted by the scientist Isaac Henry Burkill who held the position of Director of Singapore's Botanic Gardens in the early 1900s. Cloth was also saturated in a mixture of glutinous rice boiled with medicinal plants or roots. The result was a dressing similar to Elastoplast or Band-Aid. Dust left over from rice pounding went into poultices and was an excellent body rub. Lye, a powerful cleanser made from the ash of burned rice straw, was used to wash hair. After cooking the family meal, Javanese housewives still save rice water to use as a face or eye lotion.

In Java, finely-powdered rice flour is put through a lengthy fermenting process involving yeast, fungus, medicinal plants and roots such as ginger, garlic or cinnamon. It is then dried into small, round cakes that are used as the catalyst or yeast in the production of a potent, alcoholic drink.

Green Power
Kangkung (water convolvulus; *Ipomoea aquatica*), a green, leafy, water spinach beloved by Indonesians, is as important to an Indonesian menu as potatoes are in the West. It flourishes in wet, humid conditions and its pink, white and lilac flowers are often seen floating in rice paddies. *Kangkung* is awash with healthy minerals and vitamins. Leaf tips are eaten in salads, but more often the whole *kangkung* is cooked and served with

main dishes. It acts as a laxative and is recommended for piles, insomnia and headaches caused by nervousness; applying its leaves to the skin can draw out the venom from snake bites and pounded leaves are used to treat boils. The root provides a wash for haemorrhoids and is also good for white discharge, gum problems and cold sweats.

Chillies of every persuasion (*Capsicum* sp.) are found in every kitchen in Indonesia. Roughly eight kinds are regularly used in Indonesian dishes, the most popular being the finger-length red or green chilli (*cabe besar*) and the tiny, fiery bird's-eye chilli (*cabe rawit*). *Cabe besar* is used to reduce fevers and hyper-tension, and treat headaches, abdominal pains, beriberi, flu, cholera, impotence, toothache and diarrhoea; it encourages perspiration and destroys parasites. The root of *cabe rawit* is recommended for gonorrhoea and, amazingly in a tropical climate, frostbite. In Kalimantan, chilli is put into arrow poison as part of the mixture, although chilli itself contains nothing remotely poisonous. The same is true of the precisely six bird's-eye chillies that are obligatory in dyes for colouring the blade of a kris.

Chilli is used so freely in the kitchen it is rare to find a dish that escapes a few generous dollops. Fortunately, Indonesians never go short because it grows readily all over the rice fields, but is usually transplanted to a more convenient spot near the house when it matures.

Sweetcorn, Chinese mustard greens and tomatoes are eaten frequently. Sweetcorn is good for various urinary problems, mastitis and hepatitis. Chinese mustard greens treat fevers, dysentery and exhaustion. Tomatoes tackle urinary infections, the leaves relieve sunburn, while rubbing the flesh on spots can produce miraculous results. Drinking tomato juice with honey brings down fever while pure tomato juice is a cure for jaundice.

Active Desserts

Fruit is a common food in Indonesia and ideal growing conditions mean something is always ripe for dessert. The selection that follows is made on the basis of frequent and varied use as well as availability. Others, like snakefruit, which is particularly effective for diarrhoea, are harder to come by, less popular and more expensive.

Papaya (*Carica papaya*) is a fruit that crosses the divide between food, jamu and medicine. Officially it is a woody plant, but is often described as a tree. Papaya is acknowledged as a universal healer throughout Asia, especially in Indonesia where it is called the Medicine Tree. Native to Central America, the fruit was eagerly embraced by Southeast Asia's populations, and the hot, humid climate ensured papaya trees flourished in the region. Plant papaya seeds today and the tree will bear fruit just six months later.

The digestive power of papaya is well documented. In the 16th century, Columbus noted natives of the Caribbean could eat enormous meals without any sign of indigestion if papaya was served for dessert. Marco Polo believed his crew were saved from scurvy by being treated with papaya. Chester D. French, a botanist who in 1972 wrote the book *Papaya—The Melon of Health* after approximately 50 years of research on the fruit, related how an agonizing stomach cramp disappeared after a Guatemalan native gave him what he called papaya melon.

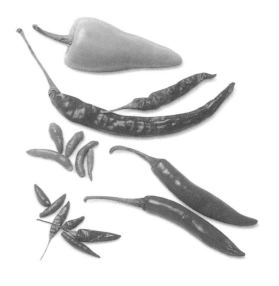

Above:
The chilli seems synonymous with Asian cuisine, so it is a surprise to find that it was introduced to tropical Asia by the Portuguese in the early 17th century.

Spanish soldiers serving with Cortez in Mexico had a similar experience. There is no doubt papaya has impressive international credentials.

It is now known that what makes the fruit so effective is an enzyme present in the juice, called papain; it seems able to digest just about anything. In its pure form papain can digest up to 35 times its own weight in lean meat, so is often used as a meat tenderiser. The enzyme is found in the juice or latex of the plant, and is highly concentrated in the leaves and skin of an unripe fruit. You only have to scratch the surface and latex flows. The pharmaceutical industry has flirted with papain for years, but its commercial potential has been hampered by the logistics of collecting and drying the latex before it rots. However, research continues because the potential profits are enormous if this problem can be overcome .

Tapping papaya requires caution. The enzyme's digestive action is so powerful that workers must avoid contact between the juice and their skin. Yet, a face mask of mashed papaya fruit will do wonders for dry, flaky skin, but it must be removed after a few minutes. A pulped paste is an effective cream for treating burns, and insect and snake bites.

Boil papaya leaves, drink the water and you'll clean the blood. To most, this is an old fashioned remedy for health, not a jamu where ingredients normally produce a chemical reaction. A mother who has problems with breastfeeding will often take papaya leaves to improve the flow and taste of her milk.

Eating papaya seeds forces out intestinal worms but beware, abortions have been caused by large doses. Over-indulge in papaya and merciless stomach cramps are the result, whilst too much papaya latex is known to inflame the intestines. Poisoners use this fact to advantage. They combine the juice with young pods from a horseradish tree, lizard egg-white and other secret ingredients to create dangerous but highly effective potions. This is not an overstatement—papaya contains active ingredients strong enough to remove the toughest warts and corns.

Papaya roots are used for tumours in the uterus, to control excessive bleeding or increase the flow of urine thus removing a kidney stone. Case histories confirm papain relieves wind, flatulence, heartburn, bad breath, bloating, headaches as well as stomach and abdominal pain. In one recorded instance, an operation for external haemorrhoids was pre-empted by papain tablets. Furthermore, papaya provides generous amounts of vitamins A and C. How much you consume and what you mix it with is obviously crucial.

Despite papaya's wonderful attributes, the plant has a few drawbacks. Mrs Kloppenburg-Versteegh, the Mrs Beaton of the Dutch East Indies (see page 16), suggests avoiding it altogether if you are hysterical, suffer from gallstones and, contrary to other opinions, have a kidney complaint. She writes that anyone suffering from eczema or women with a white discharge will itch if they persist in eating it. Her words of wisdom end with a dire warning: papaya skin should never be consumed because it contains a chemical that can cause blindness.

Unripe papaya is the key to a good *rujak* (a spicy salad of unripe fruit and vegetables) and is a favourite with West Sumatrans who fancy *urap*, a salad with coconut dressing. The young fruit can be made into jam or crystallized. If it is a bit sour, cooks boil the papaya with sugar and let it cool to make a

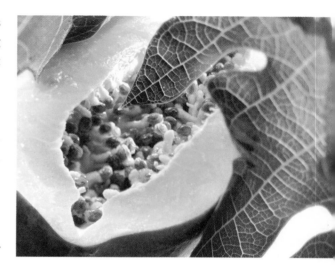

Above:
Papaya is one of the most versatile of the tropical fruits. As food it provides generous doses of vitamins A and C; as medicine it helps digestive and other health problems. Pulped papaya can also be applied to the skin where it efficiently removes blemishes like moles.

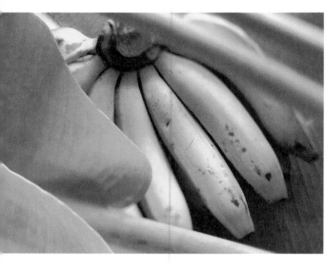

Above:
Indonesia is home to an endless choice of bananas from the sweet, stubby, dessert variety known as pisang mas *to the larger* pisang raja *and* pisang tandok, *the horn plantain used exclusively in cooking. The banana tree is useful as a source of food, medicine for intestinal complaints and fevers, whilst the leaves make instant bandages and at one time other types provided fibre for cloth.*

refreshing dessert. In Java, papaya flowers are often served as vegetables, while East Javanese half-cook the leaves and mix them with shrimp paste to produce a spicy, sambal sauce.

Never underestimate a pineapple (*Ananas* sp.). The Beverly Hills Diet made it fashionable in the West in the 1960s, and for years, top models have tucked into steak and deliberately chosen pineapple for dessert as it contains an enzyme, bromelin, that reduces meat to the consistency of porridge. In the West, pineapple juice is now recommended for thick blood and poor circulation. Again, bromelin thins the blood, prevents blood clots forming and improves blood circulation.

Originally grown in the New World, pineapples came to Asia in the 16th century courtesy of Spanish and Portuguese explorers. The Indonesian variety is smaller and sweeter than average, and grows particularly well in the red soil around Bogor, south of Jakarta. In Indonesia the fruit is traditionally eaten fresh, rubbed with salt to sweat out the juice and neutralize the acid. It comes as dessert, jam, snacks and is puréed with sugar to make drinks.

In small doses, unripe pineapple is regarded as a diuretic. Larger amounts can induce abortions because the immature fruit contains a poison that acts as a violent purge. Its young leaves are a cure for venereal disease. In the Moluccas, children drink unripe pineapple juice to remove intestinal worms and Javanese women take it to regulate menstruation.

Comprehensive as ever, Mrs Kloppenburg-Versteegh (see page 16) advised drinking the juice fresh, but never with, or straight after, milk. Experiments in a tumbler attest to its instant curdling ability. She warned kidney and diabetes patients to steer clear of pineapple and also said new mothers and women with white discharge must also avoid it. She also believed it an excellent gargle for clearing the passage to the œsophagus in cases of diphtheria.

Like papaya, the pineapple enzyme is so efficient workers in canneries have to wear gloves to protect their hands. Nonetheless Dr Jeanne Freeland-Graves, Professor of Nutrition at the University of Texas applauds pineapple as a terrific source of manganese. Apparently this is why it keeps bones strong and guards against osteoporosis.

Bananas (*pisang*; *Musa* sp.) are found and eaten everywhere in Indonesia. The country is credited with possessing 60 to 90 kinds of banana, although some argue the figure is over 100. The versatile fruit has provided Indonesians with everything from fibre for hats, matting, sewing, paper and cloth, to food, dye, *wayang* puppet stands, magic recipes, offerings in Bali and, of course, medicine. Rich in potassium, tests carried out in America reveal bananas control blood pressure and help ward off cancer of the colon if eaten before they are fully ripe.

Young banana leaves come in handy for dressing wounds, and their cooling effect makes them suitable for treating eye diseases. The juice is an antidote to diarrhoea and excessive bleeding during menstruation. The Balinese dry and pound banana skins into flour, and boil the stem with spices to make a vegetable dish called *ares*. Bananas can be a gargle, remedy for angina and a tonic for stimulating hair growth. But it all depends on which banana.

Juice from the stem of *pisang kepok* or *pisang klutuk* is used to treat snake bites, kidney stones and bleeding following delivery. Once upon a time fruit from the *pisang klutuk* was burnt in

Kalimantan Standbys

Project Barito Ulu is a scientific research programme set up to determine the most effective way of conserving and regenerating rainforests. Bapak Suriantata, a member of the Barito team, who was born in Kalimantan and has used traditional medicine all his life, passed on some first-hand experiences.

Remedies from his province are largely made from tree bark, he says. "Bark from the young coconut tree, nutmeg, fenugreek (*keci beling*; *Sericocalyx crispus*), *meniran* also known as *gendong anak* (*Phyllanthus niruri*; 'the child pick-a-back', so called owing to the fruit's position on the back of tree branches) and cat's whiskers (*Orthosiphon aristatus*; *kumis kuching*) are mixed together as a treatment for kidney stones. A blocked nose can be easily cleared by scraping wet bark from the cinnamon tree and placing it on the bridge of the nose. If my daughter suffers from stomach pain or dysentery, I get some guava seeds, grind them up, add water and leave them to steep. When the brew is strong enough I give her one teaspoon morning and night until she recovers. As soon as the symptoms disappear she stops taking the medicine."

kitchen ash and pressed to obtain the juice, which was given to dysentery patients. To avoid such a tedious process, the alternative was to add a pinch of saffron and some opium to the astringent juice and swallow it down. By contrast, *pisang swanggi* is an antidote for poison, while on the islands of Ambon and Ceram, cooked *pisang tunjuk* is a diuretic. Uncooked *tunjuk* results in unbearable itching and red urine.

The National Heart Institute of America found bananas contained serotonin, which activates the smooth muscle of the intestine and is also useful for depression and migraine. Another of its substances, norepinephrine, helps in certain cases of heart collapse. But beware the not-so-desirable side effects of bananas other than *pisang mas*, golden bananas. They have the property to increase wetness in the vagina, which, according to most Indonesian herbalists, is not an attribute the average Indonesian husband is happy about.

Other Common Curative Ingredients

There is a plethora of other fruits and vegetables that are almost equally important. Indonesians have taken advantage of their resources and developed an impressive number of medicines—both preventative and curative—from their store cupboard.

One example, the giant white radish (*Raphanus sativus*; *lobak*) takes care of fluid retention. Another, the sour, fragrant juice of yellow thin-skinned lime (*Citrus aurantifolia*; *jeruk nipis*) appears in numerous recipes from sauces and marinades to fish and meat dishes. It has the ability to detoxify poisons in the body and is added to many jamu, especially those prescribed for diarrhoea and sore throats. *Jeruk nipis* even finds its way into compresses.

Isaac Henry Burkill notes no less than 29 remedies are known to contain *jeruk nipis*, partly for its therapeutic value and partly because it acts as a carrier, but particularly because it puts paid to evil spirits.

Coconut, perhaps the most widely used of tropical fruits, is renowned for treating dysentery. Indonesians combine the old leaves of the cashew nut and other ingredients to treat burns and skin diseases. The cashew nut, however, is more usually seen as food rather than medicine.

To gauge what is meant by medicinal food in Indonesia, take a look at familiar items used by cooks in Bali and Java. Given their availability, most of us would not recognize them as curing, let alone know which parts to use or what to do with them. For example red onions can be prescribed for anything from fluid retention, sleeplessness and reducing fever in children, to treating diabetes, helping menstruation problems, dysentery and colic. The universal healer, garlic, is regarded as good for wind, water retention, reducing phlegm, paralysis, hypertension and purifying the blood. White pepper apparently works well as a contraceptive, relieves wind and water retention, stops vomiting and is a remedy for leprosy and eczema.

In Indonesia, there are thousands of recipes and methods to prepare these healing foods. A detailed analysis would fill volumes, particularly as many foods are recommended for the same ailment. For example, papaya and pineapple are said to aid good digestion. Our purpose here is to show that food contributes to good health, rather than to provide exhaustive lists. And in Indonesia, as we see, the lines blur between healing foods, health-giving foods and traditional medicine.

A Horticultural Expert

H. J. Abdul Talib (see opposite, bottom) is a horticulturalist who specializes in growing plants and trees used in traditional medicine. He is a highly respected member of Koperasie Jamu Tradisional Mugi Rakit, Yogyakarta (an association whose name translates as "wishing to see unanimous agreement") whose knowledge is frequently sought by medical experts.

Over the past 20 years, Pak Talib and his wife have established a small but outstanding example of a Family Medicinal Garden or FAME (see opposite, top). In response to a recommendation from the World Health Organization, urging developing countries to make full use of their natural medical resources, the Indonesian Government has been encouraging the cultivation of FAMEs in every village so families can make effective traditional drugs cheaply in their own homes.

Long term, the Government see such gardens supporting a wide range of activities from reforestation, nature preservation and eradication of communicable diseases, to growing healthy, nutritious food. They want villagers to make extra income by developing FAMEs and growing raw, natural drugs for sale to industry—particularly drug manufacturers— through cooperative stores. The idea is particularly relevant where plants and roots are used only in small quantities or are difficult to grow.

The Talibs, both tertiary educated, are totally committed to the scheme's success and see themselves as pioneers. Their garden measures approximately 30 square metres (100 square feet) and within this relatively small area are some 4,000 plants. Its maintenance is an endless, back-breaking task for the whole family, including the Talib's three sons.

The family sell plants and leaves, but do not make medicines. However, to encourage customers to grow their own remedies, they give each one a bonus of fresh ginger leaves which cannot be found in local markets.

"People come to us precisely because we can supply plants that are impossible to buy anywhere else. We stay open 24 hours because customers often turn up at 11pm or midnight. But business isn't our prime concern. Our real work is to conserve important plants and persuade jamu makers to expand their repertoire by using barks and leaves as well as the standard roots and tubers."

Among the inventory is *cimera* (also known as *jahe merah* or red ginger; *Zingiber officinale* var. *rubrum*), a rare plant indigenous to Kalimantan and the Moluccas, but not found on Java. Combined with other ingredients and made into a paste, the result is a proven remedy for skin complaints and sprains; *jeruk kingkit* (lime berry; *Triphasia trifolia*) is boiled up with loaf sugar to make cough syrup; the dried or fresh leaves of *kumis kuching* (cat's whiskers; *Orthosiphon aristatus*) which grow in profusion can increase the flow of urine.

"We've tried to include a wide variety of hard trees in this garden," Pak Talib explains. "Most growers only cultivate herbs and plants but we believe hard trees are very important in traditional medicine. We try to plant the complete range of ingredients for natural medicine, no matter how difficult or how large."

Pak Talib also has the distinction of owning a white Java Plum tree (*duwet*). Such trees are almost impossible to cultivate and are consequently very rare. The white Java Plum tree fruit is usually taken with coffee and is famous for treating diabetes. The black fruit, on the other hand, is also an excellent cure for diabetes; it is wonderful to eat, very sweet and widely available.

A special section has been created for classical plants, a term applied to plants traditionally grown in the palace grounds. In this category Pak Talib is justifiably proud of his *kepel* trees (*Stelechocarpus burahol*). "The fruit removes the smell of urine or underarm odour, and also tastes delicious," he says.

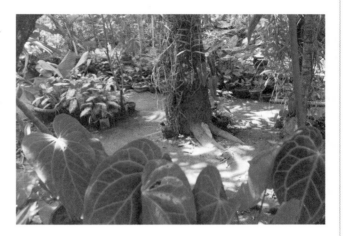

Adjoining the classical garden is a special layout of herbs and plants specially grown to the requirements of Dr Sulis from the Public Health Service Centre in Yogyakarta. Pak Talib's design worked so well that it has been adopted as the model for the city and surrounding area.

A pragmatist at heart, Pak Talib has an ingenious solution to combat the increasing lack of space as Java's population expands—to grow important medicinal trees and shrubs as bonsai miniatures. "They are decorative, space-saving, absorb weather pollution and provide fresh ingredients for making jamu and other remedies," he asserts. He has already produced a *jerek kingkip* bonsai and successfully experimented with boiling up its red berries to make cough mixture. Tamarind, too, has been dwarfed and work is progressing on other specimens.

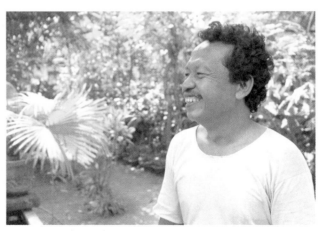

The Talib plants represent over 1,000 varieties, which they claim provide the necessary materials for 52 different traditional medicines. While most growers fight shy of the rare or delicate species, Pak Talib enjoys the challenge of nurturing them from propagation to maturity. He insists that "problem plants don't exist—every plant is easy to grow".

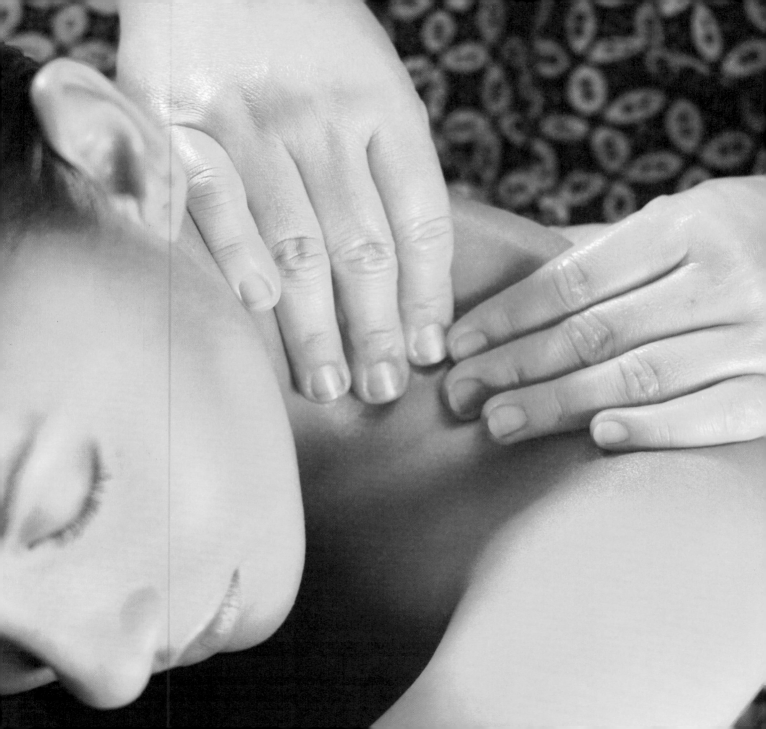

Chapter 4. Massage: The Power of Touch

Massage is an integral part of the Indonesian approach to inner and outer health and beauty.

Left:
Massage is an integral part of Indonesian inner and outer health and beauty. Here, the masseuse uses a 'pinching' technique where the flesh is pulled up between the thumb and forefingers.

Massage is an integral part of the Indonesian approach to inner and outer health and beauty. Records existing from Ancient Rome to India, and from Egypt to Indonesia indicate that the curing power of massage has been known for centuries, even millennia. Some of the first instances of using hands in health care can be found in records dating back over 15,000 years. Massage in its various different forms has been documented on papyrus scrolls, old manuscripts and rock carvings throughout the world, including the famous stone reliefs of Borobudur, the 8th–9th century Buddhist stupa in Central Java.

It is thought that early medicine relied heavily on massage. Massage techniques were studied as part of classical Greek medicine, and the laying on of hands and massage were an important element in early Christian healing, until the church decided that anything connected with the body was sinful. The erotic overtones of massage ensured it was one of the first casualties of this new thinking. It was not until the evolution of what we now call Swedish massage, by Henri Peter Ling (in Sweden he is known as Per Heinrik Ling), a student at Stockholm University in the early 1800s, that massage regained respectability in Europe.

Hotelier Turner Healer

Pak Hadi may not have had an orthodox training as a masseur and healer, but his knowledge garners results. Trained in hotel management, this hotelier turned healer lives in the outskirts of Solo, where he receives patients. In his garden he grows medicinal herbs, trees and shrubs to replenish his apothecary, each item meticulously tagged with its scientific name. Thirty kilometres (18 miles) outside Solo he also maintains a considerably larger herbal garden, with the help of four full-time workers.

Pak Hadi has had considerable success treating cancer patients, diabetes sufferers and people with kidney complaints, using reflexology combined with herbal preparations and healing techniques. Out of the 29,000 people who have visited his clinic, he has been able to cure a number of patients of supposedly incurable cancer through a combination of jamu and reflexology. Breast cancer patients are cured using papaya roots; liver cancer with *daun dewa* (*Gynura procumbens*) and prostate and bone cancer with a mixture of ingredients from his garden. Medical sceptics, he reveals, have been known to come to his practice under the guise of requiring a check-up, to see his techniques for themselves. One such patient was a female doctor who he discovered was suffering from cervical cancer. He offered to treat her but she preferred Western methods.

Pak Hadi mentions there are over 1,300 medicinal plants, but his formulæ for jamu rely largely on the use of some 34 major herbs. From these he distills 18 main types of jamu and uses them in 300 to 500 different mixtures. As he points out, many herbs and plants are readily available in Indonesian markets, but unless the jamu maker has complete knowledge of how to both prepare and administer them correctly, they will be ineffective. He is pictured below practising reflexology on a patient.

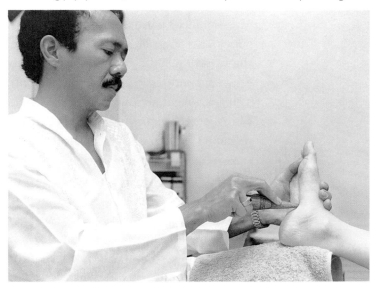

In the East, belief in the healing touch never wavered. During the T'ang Dynasty, AD 618–907, the Chinese Imperial Medical Bureau had a special Department of Massage. In 8th-century Japan, the Nara Medical College included massage courses in its curriculum, while in India, Ayurvedic lymphatic massage was a permanent feature of family life. Once established, these techniques flourished—and continue to flourish—in Asia.

Having come under the influence of China, India and Arabia, Indonesians observed and selected massage techniques and created their own unique style. Elements of acupressure, pressure point massage, shiatsu and reflexology can be clearly identified in most Indonesian treatments. Relatively recently, Swedish massage has been introduced to the country as an increasing number of Indonesians train overseas. However, among the old school masseurs, the term 'Swedish massage' is often derogatory and used to describe the efforts of a masseur who has learned skills in a school rather than by apprenticeship or hands-on experience. True Swedish massage does exist but the newcomer to massage treatments ought to determine exactly what type of massage is being offered before treatment.

Massage in Indonesia

Massage comes from the Greek *massein*, to knead, and the Arabic *mass*, to press gently. For the Westerner, the word conjures up images of aromatic oils and rhythmic movement, lulling mind and body into a sense of warmth and security. This notion corresponds with the idea of a Western Swedish massage, whose goal is to tone and relax the body or assist healing in sport-induced injuries. However, this is not what the average

Indonesian understands by massage. Massage in Indonesia is usually associated with helping the body rid itself of disease, regain its inherent health, and ensure an on-going state of good health. Indonesian massage experts happily use methods that would horrify their Western counterparts, though their techniques can effectively remove the appearance of varicose veins and other undesirables.

Two traditional types of massage are practised: *pijat* and *urut*. The word *pijat* means massage in Indonesian, while *urut* means massage in Javanese. *Pijat* is the ubiquitous massage (it is also the name for a masseur), and is very relaxing. In its most basic form, it is known as *cape*, a massage that is widely practised in the village and consists of a simple, repetitive squeezing movement of the flesh between the fingers and palm of the hand. *Urut* is more specialized and is usually used for the treatment of bone fractures. *Urut* treatments are considered *halus*, meaning refined or smooth: fluidity and gentleness are the hallmarks of this massage.

Training and Work

Massage skills are usually passed from master to pupil, although in Java it is also taught at centres set up to promote traditional healing and massage, encourage correct technique, and enhance understanding of the therapy. Martina Berto and Mustika Ratu have begun such official massage courses. A student can expect to master basic massage skills in three to six weeks, but must enrol in a year's course for *pijat* or *urut*. At grassroots level, the elderly *pijat* (masseur) 'trains' a student using an intuitive method. Tips, such as the types of illness that do not

Pak Karto's Mission

When only 15 years of age, Pak Karto decided to make helping people his life's work. When he saw how massage and reflexology relieved pain, he recognized that these disciplines could be his tools. The youngster's enthusiasm persuaded a local doctor to take the boy under his wing and thus his 55-year career began. Today, over 70 years of age, he has the confidence of someone who knows his business thoroughly.

"Men or women—it doesn't matter," he says. "I've learnt the anatomy and physiology of both and know exactly where to massage more gently. I can tell immediately if someone is healthy or sick from the state of their blood circulation." He then adds: "Bad blood circulation causes many problems (even toothache) and massage is effective in these circumstances. Treatment varies; tiredness can be sorted out quickly but serious conditions take longer because you have to work extra carefully." His ability to see beyond superficial symptoms is uncanny, but Pak Karto regards it as normal diagnosis.

"Patients usually know they're ill," affirms Pak Karto, "But they often have no idea why. That's where my training comes in. I often get to the root of the trouble when other methods fail." In one memorable case, a 10-year old boy, unable to walk, was brought to the masseur. He was able to untangle the child's nerves through massage, and the boy was cured.

Prayer is not part of the treatment, but in his mind Pak Karto always asks God's help before every massage. While other masseurs use oils to move the hands over the patient's body, Pak Karto does not, and in fact prefers the patient to remain fully clothed. "Oil actually hampers me," he reveals, "It makes the skin too soft and slippery, and I can't feel the body properly. Oil rarely has anything to do with pain or sickness. It's the inside that counts."

Day or night, anyone arriving on Pak Karto's doorstep will be helped. His is a large brick house with concrete floors, a sign of wealth in Central Java. Despite his affluence, Pak Karto prefers the simple life. The house and his black and white television are exceptions. "Family pressure was mounting so eventually I caved in over the television," he explains with an embarrassed smile.

"I believe that enough is OK, that's my motto in life. With enough you are always happy." He warms to this theme: "If you're rich, you keep wanting more and more money and spend your life worrying you'll lose it. This is what breeds unhappiness." For this reason, and like all genuine massage experts, he doesn't have a fixed charge, but operates on something akin to the Robin Hood principle: the more wealthy patients subsidize the less well-off.

Pak Karto has a particularly hectic lifestyle because he continues to work at a local timber yard and, despite earning more through massage, has no plans to give up this regular work. This leaves him little time to relax; even in the evening, after he has slipped into a traditional sarong, clients still turn up.

"It's always the same, no sooner have I settled myself comfortably than a patient springs up out of the blue," he says, "But then I'm never really content unless I'm helping someone."

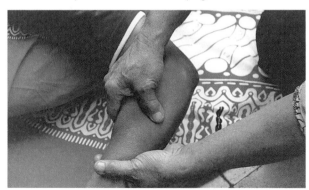

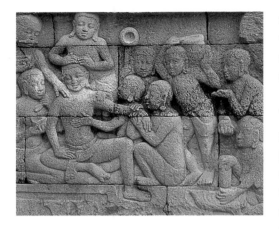

respond well to massage; when massage should not be used; and when a masseur should not work, are given. But at both levels, regular arm and finger exercises are advocated, as these prevent the masseur from becoming quickly tired whilst working.

Both men and women may train to become expert therapists. Women, who are known as *Ibu pijat*, tend to work mainly in people's homes, while men are more likely to set up a group practice. Blind massage experts are believed to be best, as lack of sight is thought to heighten their sense of touch; furthermore, the delicate questions regarding modesty are by-passed. Thanks to the massage courses run by Jakarta's School for the Blind, the services of such massage experts are still available.

In Indonesia, massage establishments range from small, run-down shops to large salons; from joints where a cursory oily rub leads to sex, to dedicated clinics with highly skilled therapists. An example of the latter is the Puri Ayu salon owned by famous jamu-producer, Martha Tilaar. Although prices are far from budget, the results are worth the investment. Outside major towns, where the emphasis is on health; people often weigh up the cost of visiting a doctor, who may be more than a couple of hours' journey away, and often plump for a massage instead. A good masseur commands enormous respect and status in a community.

Above:
Stone reliefs at the most famous of Javan stupas, Borobudur, depict a massage taking place.

The Technique

Practitioners of both *pijat* and *urut* massage often begin by saying a silent prayer or repeating a mantra asking for the recovery of their patient and seeking God's help. The ritual gives both patient and healer a psychological boost and reinforces the masseur's belief in her curing ability. Her next task is to transfer this strength to the patient's body by either rubbing or shaking her hands over it. It is believed that energy fields inside and surrounding the body may be changed through prayer, which in turn may affect a person's health.

The patient lies face down on a hard surface, usually the floor, while the masseur works her way from legs to head, back and front, belching loudly as she goes. The reason for this practice? *Pijat* practitioners of the old school are convinced they draw wind out of the patient's body through their fingers. To avoid absorbing the sickness themselves, they then must burp to get rid of it, and encourage patients to do likewise.

Both *pijat* and *urut* massage have precise technical terms that differentiate between the movements in a sequence. These movements are poles apart even if the two approaches are similar. *Pijat* generally works on the muscles—a masseur uses her own routine and utilizes medium to strong kneading and squeezing. *Urut*, on the other hand, goes much deeper and works on the muscles and nerve path. Thus, this healing massage involves some fairly tough pressing and beating on specific points which can be uncomfortable at times. Its main purpose is to encourage smooth blood circulation.

In *pijat*, the fingers hold an area being worked on while the thumb produces a pressured squeeze. The muscles may also be pulled up very slowly using all the fingers, while a different technique involves three fingers moving in an anti-clockwise, circular motion. 'Big' and 'small' pinching is done between the middle and index fingers. Small pinching pulls little muscles, such as those hidden in the armpit.

Massage Remedies Limp

Tom Nayoan, finance consultant and publisher, had difficulty walking. He assumed spending hours in the car was responsible and concluded he must live with stiffness, pain and a lopsided gait. That was before masseuse Ibu Ana was consulted and diagnosed the muscles on one leg as being totally intertwined. As she gradually released and returned them to their correct position, Tom couldn't believe the change.

"I've had massage for years," he complained, "But clearly they didn't know what they were doing." He is now out of pain for the first time in months and walking normally.

Urut incorporates some of the movements used in *pijat* but is more intense and demands additional skills. To cure successfully, *urut* practitioners must know nerve, acupuncture or pressure points. Thumbs, fingers, knuckles, fist, palm and body weight are all used. This form of massage hits muscles below the surface and utilizes its own sets of movements. Thumb pressure, or *jempol*, is a series of small, short, press-and-pull movements along a straight line holding the thumb upright; *unceg* is a similar technique but the thumb is held at 45 degrees. Typical movements include forming a 'V' shape between fingers and thumb, or locking thumbs together to create extra strength. *Tiga jari* is another movement employing three fingers, pressing upwards at 60 to 75 degrees from the patient's body. A variation duplicates the press-and-pull thumb action but uses three fingers. Using the palm and five fingers in a circular, squeezing motion on the calf, buttocks and shoulder is yet another approach known as *ramas*, as is *desar telapak*, a technique of holding the arm at 60 to 75 degrees and working only with the palm. Each set of movements is highly specialized.

Sorting out Problems

The masseur works with different points and varies her routine to suit each patient. For example, *urut* restores muscle tone, helps to heal broken bones and removes toxins by stimulating the lymphatic system. The massage also improves sexual vitality and encourages the growth of new cells, which keeps the body looking firmer and younger. Impotence is treated with short thumb presses on the sole of a foot near the heel; cases of acute insomnia are helped by pressing three points on the head.

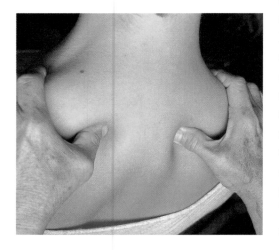

Above:
When thumb pressure is applied to certain areas of the body, the masseur does not hold back. The patient may feel some initial pain, but results override any discomfort.

Massage for high blood pressure starts at the head; if low, on the back. Manipulation in *urut* can be painful, but if done skillfully may sort out minor problems, like a stiff neck, in one swift movement. Acupuncture points are useful targets during this massage as pressure on such points may benefit ailments in another part of the body.

Choosing the appropriate massage for the patient is all-important. The gentler style of *pijat* is unlikely to help severely twisted muscles. Such injuries need time and tougher measures. Western studies have already proved back massage heightens activity of the sympathetic nervous system, thereby increasing blood pressure, pulse, respiration and skin temperature without putting strain on the heart. An *urut* expert would be well aware of these anatomical factors, whereas the average *pijat* masseur would not. *Urut* massage is precise and highly technical and bearing with the initial discomfort is worthwhile. The feeling of well-being after a good *urut* massage is indescribable. Backache, stress, aching shoulders, tense muscles and headaches fade away. The biggest bonus for many women is that cellulite melts away after six to eight sessions. You may feel drained and sleepy after the initial shock to the system, but following a few one to two hour appointments, you'll be dozing off during treatment. It is a most relaxing experience.

Massage releases endorphins—the body's equivalent of morphine—into the system, and this may make a client crave another treatment. While a light daily massage cannot do any harm, once the body is toned and healthy no more than two healing massages per week are recommended, because excessive massage is counter-productive. Clients who become addicted

Coping with a Tropical Climate

When Sue Burden first arrived in Indonesia, she could not tolerate the tropical climate. Unusually heavy perspiration, exhaustion and pain in her legs and hips made going out a major task. This would be a handicap for many, but for a photographer it spelt disaster.

Over two years she tried dozens of prescription drugs, to no avail. Finally, she decided to try traditional healing, and braved a two-hour drive, early one morning, to the Puncak mountains to see Pak Haji Asyhar Fauzi.

She arrived at his clinic where up to 600 patients are seen each Sunday. The wait lasted hours, but she was finally shown into the treatment room, where Pak Haji treated her to "deep scratching" on her feet, knees, lower back and neck. Pak Haji then dressed each scratch. Later at home, Sue found the only signs of her visit to the Puncak healer were a few marks on the most sensitive areas, which cleared up the following day. Within two days, Sue reported feeling 80 per cent better.

Three weeks later, the symptoms started to return, so Sue set out for a second visit, this time armed with a doctor's report stating she had low blood pressure. Pak Haji welcomed this Western diagnosis and repeated his earlier performance. This time Sue announced she felt all but cured. By the time she left Indonesia two months later, her health had improved enormously. Ask Pak Haji what method he uses and he points upwards, saying, "It's nothing to do with me—I just let God guide my hands—it's his work, not mine."

Pressure Point Therapy

Pak Herri is a healer who relies primarily on massage, assisted by jamu. Pinching, squeezing, pressing and 'knuckle dusting' are the techniques employed by the team of four experts at his casual and friendly practice in South Jakarta. A massage will last between 15 to 30 minutes, depending on the illness and its severity, but patients may have to wait several hours before their treatment even begins.

The masseur sits beside the patient turned towards the feet and works his way up the pressure points on the calves, occasionally stretching an arm behind him to include the thigh area. Then he turns around completely to tackle the buttocks, back and shoulders. The procedure is repeated three times with varying degrees of intensity. If the client is fit, there is no pain.

According to Pak Herri's training chart, there are 34 pressure points on the legs, six around the feet, six over the chest and eleven on the neck and face. The massage focuses on the calves because they account for nearly half the body's pressure points: 26 out of 57. The remainder of the treatment is centred on the back, shoulders, neck and head with a little work on the feet— and a resounding toe-cracking finish. The practice makes its own special cream from fresh ginger, which is applied to the calves and the small of the back. It feels hot and allows the masseur to go in deeper without inflicting additional pain.

Pak Herri explains that the body is equipped with a complete range of chemical substances. As long as the body functions normally, each substance performs its job as nature intended. However, if the circulation stops working properly and toxins are not eliminated from the system, a whole chain of adverse chemical reactions occur.

"Anything can happen," says Pak Herri cheerfully, "cholesterol or uric acid levels can rise, cancer or diabetes may develop—you just can't tell. Our technique is designed to look after circulation and is especially effective for treating the heart, lungs

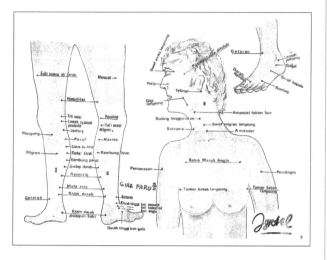

and feet. We've had excellent results with Hepatitis B if it's caught in the early stages and my own speciality is heart bypass patients. Very often I can open up the arteries with massage, which allows the heart to work normally again, removing any need for surgery."

Pak Herri is a firm believer in following nature's way and has various rules for good health. Rule 1 is to follow a regular exercise programme; rule 2 is to consume copious amounts of room-temperature water and rule 3 is to avoid cold drinks, ice and air-conditioning. Why is avoiding the cold so important? Because cold stops the body perspiring and toxins can't escape.

"I often see patients who are suffering from cramp because they've been swimming in cold water. Westerners are the worst offenders. They come to the tropics and use every means they can to stay cool, when in fact it's the last thing they should be doing. Interfering with nature in this way never does any good."

can end up damaging their muscles, which become flabby. Furthermore, sensitive areas like the feet can become very sore from excessive massage. By the third or fourth session with a *pijat* masseur, the pain practically disappears. The masseur has beaten most of the knots and bumps into submission and thereafter the body only needs a regular maintenance programme.

In many cases, the masseur's job does not stop at massage. If he is from the traditional school, his instincts for your well being will be holistic and he will hand out advice on diet and herbal medicine, never doubting that it will be followed. This is yet another example of the overlap between jamu and healing. Generally, older, more experienced *pijat* masseurs give better massages. But the most important thing is to develop a good rapport between you and your masseur, or results may be disappointing. Like doctors, dentists or hairdressers, you must have faith in the masseur's abilities. If not, you should find another.

What is the magic formula for diagnosis? Masseurs say they can tell if something is wrong when an area hurts, the skin turns red or they feel a hard lump. Most ask clients if they are sick and draw on knowledge built up over years. Good masseurs have a highly developed sense of touch and identify peculiarities by comparing their client's body with the norm. While massage can relieve and cure numerous aches and pains, it cannot fight fevers such as malaria.

There are many massage techniques and theories. For example, M'Bok Na is self taught and comes from Central Java. She massages the left side of the body very thoroughly, especially the back, believing that the whole back benefits from intense work on one side. By the time she moves over to the other side,

Fixing a Damaged Knee

John Herbert slipped while dashing down a ramp in the pouring rain, and felt something snap. At the doctor's surgery, he was given an impressive array of pills, but they did not work. When he consulted an orthopaedic specialist in Singapore, he was advised to swim and work out on an exercise bike. Three weeks later, however, John found he could hardly walk. It was at this point someone he knew recommended visiting Pak Haji Naim, a renowned bone expert who owns a clinic in South Jakarta.

First the *patah tulang* examined the knee and carefully assessed the damage. He then applied a heavy, oily cream, made on the premises, to the affected area and began to massage it. Within five minutes, John could "actually feel the bits of splintered bone being pushed back where they belonged". The rubbing continued for another ten minutes, after which pads of cotton wool soaked in oil were applied above, below and round the knee. Finally, tiny bamboo splints measuring about 2 x 10 cm (1 x 4 in) were placed over the swollen part of the knee and bound tightly in place with an elastic bandage.

John was then asked to test his leg. The improvement was immediately evident: he could put more weight on it than when he arrived. Three half-half hour visits later, John could walk again, albeit a little stiffly. By the time he returned to the USA, even though his knee had not healed completely, doctors said that without Pak Haji Naim's intervention the problem might have become permanent.

the job is more or less done, with only a light massage left to wrap it up. In sharing M'bok's theory with Professor Dr Sardjono, he said: "She's right. If one side of the body is put in order there is a knock-on effect and treating the other one is much easier." Strength is adjusted to suit the patient; they must feel the pressure but it should not be unbearable. Thumb pressure is used for light massage while the three-fingered action, palms and pinching fall into the medium bracket. Anything else is considered hard.

Cupping

The use of cupping-glasses in healing is tedious, troublesome and somewhat inconvenient. In essence, a heated glass or cup is placed on the skin; as it cools, the blood below is drawn to the surface, and this is said to improve circulation. It creates a hot, biting sensation on the skin which is not painful. Today, the technique is practised in Indonesia, China, Indochina and, interestingly, in parts of France. Indonesia has seen a decline in cupping though the technique still enjoys some success with the older generation. Their children prefer jamu or Western medicine. Most Westerners regard cupping as a relic from the Dark Ages (when indeed it was one of the most popular medical treatments) and are vague about its purpose.

In Java, cupping techniques take on complicated overtones. A small amount of coconut oil is poured into a ceramic saucer, which is placed directly onto the stomach or back. A piece of cloth or cotton wool is set alight on the oil, creating a makeshift candle. A larger upturned glass or cup is placed completely over the saucer where lack of oxygen makes it stick to the skin. After about 15 minutes, a red mark appears where blood has been brought to the surface. The whole tiresome business is repeated wherever there is pain. Older Javanese swear by it for removing the ever-present 'wind'.

Money Massage
Called *kerokan*, this technique can make a patient look as if he has been viciously attacked. A coin is dragged diagonally across the skin, leaving livid red lines as the masseur works on the back, neck, shoulders, backside, stomach, and sometimes feet. *Kerokan* is painless if correctly administered.

Most *kampung* people living traditional lifestyles, particularly in North Java, utilize *kerokan* to alleviate colds and colic. According to Indonesian belief, it expels bad wind from the body: wind (known as *masuk angin*) embraces a host of illnesses from feeling unwell, tired, weak or stiff to aching bones, pins and needles or the common cold. But in all cases the root cause is seen as abnormal blood circulation or malfunctioning red blood cells, a problem *kerokan* alleviates very successfully. If a medical doctor diagnoses wind—or gas—in the abdomen, *kerokan* is often recommended to relieve the nausea and discomfort. This is because it encourages the patient to belch thus, it is said, removing any impurities.

Pregnancy and Post-Natal Care
Ante-natal massage is popular in Indonesia. Regular massage helps relieve pregnancy pains, promotes blood circulation, relieves water retention, and encourages relaxation. Every two weeks during the last two months of pregnancy, Javanese

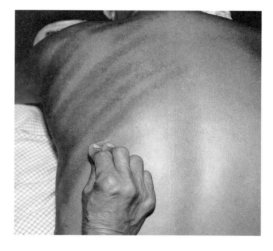

Above:
Kerokan *massage is practised by pulling a coin diagonally down the skin, leaving livid red lines behind. Surprisingly, it is not in the least painful.*

Massage Pointers from an Expert

Ibu Evelyn, one-time employee of the Department of Health Education and physiotherapist to the Indonesian Olympic team, is an experienced masseuse with considerable training in alternative medicines. She not only studied in Indonesia but took time out to learn the ancient traditions of acupuncture, reflexology and pressure point massage in Hong Kong and Taiwan.

She cites today's lifestyle as a factor in many complaints. "People make themselves ill," Ibu Evelyn says. "The trouble usually begins on the inside; stress builds up slowly. It can literally take years before it shows up as sickness. That's why you can't fix the problem overnight. It's not like a strained muscle." Massage, she explains, is the best way to combat stress as it relaxes the body and stimulates circulation. Blood circulation is the body's distribution system and thus essential for good health.

"When a patient feels the body getting warm during massage it's a sign the circulation is improving," she adds. But Ibu Evelyn recognizes that some complaints are not apparent on the surface. "Hardness is a common sign of trouble but you need to look out for tension, red skin and compare symptoms with those of other clients. The masseuse must also be careful not to press too hard unless someone is strong and healthy, otherwise muscles become inflamed or strained. Watch out for fair skin because it is also more fragile and usually turns red during a tough massage." "Normally," she adds, "it's only friction bringing blood to the surface and there's no cause for alarm."

Developing her own technique, Ibu Evelyn combines scientific principles with traditional Indonesian massage, acupressure-acupuncture and reflexology. Her bias towards reflexology came about because "it works directly on the nerves and is holistic; by pressing reflex points on the feet, you treat the whole body".

Ibu Evelyn believes that successful massage comes down to skilled handwork. "Let the body dictate, then supply what it needs" is her advice. Illnesses differ, people differ and the right blend of strokes must be chosen for each patient. For example, pressure points are not always found in the same place. "You can't follow a massage routine willy nilly," is the warning. "You have to use your brain." Oils are governed by the same rule, she says. "They must suit the patient. I would never mix an oil without first checking the whole body, particularly the skin. Rough skin benefits from heavy oil and Minyak Tawon is a good all-purpose oil. I mix it with skin cream which also softens the skin; other oils can be used straight from the bottle."

Although Ibu Evelyn has retired from teaching, she is still involved with Indonesian massage. She has penned two books aimed at upgrading and standardizing massage practice. She would like to see a more scientific approach to massage and hopes that one day she will create a massage training school. For the moment, however, that remains a project in the pipeline.

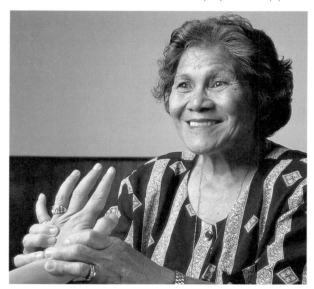

women drink half a glass of freshly-made coconut oil laced with herbs, which is said to ease and speed up the delivery. Even today, Indonesian women normally give birth in less than four hours as opposed to the average eight to 16 for a Caucasian, but it is difficult to tell whether this is due to physiology, jamu or massage, or a combination of all three.

The technique of post-natal massage is one of Indonesia's secrets. Although this knowledge has strayed across neighbouring borders, it remains the exclusive property of the Indonesian-Malay community. What is known, however, is that the mother regains her looks, health and strength within 30 to 40 days of the baby's arrival. Treatments are usually carried out by elderly, experienced masseurs, who fully understand the concept of inner and outer beauty their clients strive to achieve.

The post-natal *Ibu pijat* begins work in the early morning when her client washes in hot, instead of cold, water. While the mother is bathing, the masseuse prepares charcoal in a pot burner. Following her bath, the mother spends 15 minutes standing over the burning charcoal to warm her body and tighten the vaginal muscles. Next comes a herbal oil body massage to restore muscle tone. This is followed by pulling the mother's hair back tightly to remove wind and relieve migraines or headaches. At this stage, a poultice is applied to the stomach. Cajuput oil, juice of the thin-skinned lime and *kapur sirih*— a mixture of lime powder and betel leaves—are mixed with *tapel* powder to form a paste. This cleans out any blood remaining in the womb, firms the muscles and shrinks the stomach. Such precautions counteract stomach ache and help the mother regain her figure.

Below:
*Binding is a common
post-natal treatment in
Indonesia helping a
new mother firm up her
muscles and regain her
figure in less than one
month.*

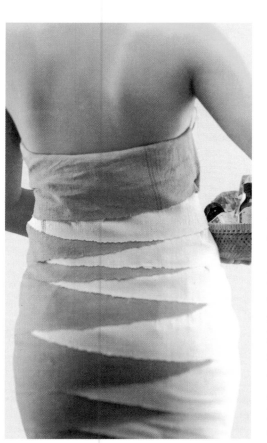

If the birth was normal the *Ibu pijat* pushes up the womb to prevent the woman from becoming pregnant again too easily. Finally the binding is put in place. Before modern medicine developed ways of stitching tears in the vaginal opening following delivery, the skin was pulled together and bound, enabling it to heal more quickly, provided the mother didn't move her legs too far apart and cause the skin to tear again.

The binding, *bengkung* in Javanese, resembles an adult form of swaddling, except it is wound from the hips to the rib cage. It is made of hard, cotton cloth measuring anything from eight to 15 metres (25 feet to 45 feet) in length, and is often bound in a 'V' shape over the stomach for extra strength. To achieve its objective, the binding needs to be unbearably tight. The swaddling requires a mother to sleep with her legs straight out in front of her and keep as still as possible. Possibly the worst aspect if one lives in the tropics is being unable to shower for 24 hours. The mother can only bathe when her masseur undoes the cloth each morning. In the old days, these bindings were uncomfortably hot as there were no fans or air-conditioning.

Jamu was an integral part of this procedure. Nowadays Indonesians buy new mothers a prettily packaged gift set containing all the mixtures and pills needed for her confinement. For instance the Mustika Ratu set includes Tapel Raket Mustika Sejati to cleanse the womb and Minyak Kayu Putih for stomach ache plus Bubuk Bancar Air Susu, a powder that works in tandem with Jamu Galian Parem Wangi to ensure the quality and flow of a mother's milk. This is important because Indonesian mothers sometimes breastfeed their children up to the age of three or four years.

Parem Segar Sumyah is another remedy for new mothers. It is a hard, powder tablet to which warm water and *gandapura* oil are added. Rubbing this liquid onto the body is supposed to make it young and healthy again. For external care, Pilis Wangi is a compress to make the eyes bright and shiny. Jamu Pulih Balung Sumsum—health-restoring pills made from marrow—are taken with warm water in the afternoons to ward off tiredness or aches and pains. For the baby, there is one small bottle of Minyak Telon for rubbing on the skin after bathing. Theoretically this oil protects the child against wind and other minor ailments.

Post-natal treatment today remains much the same as in the past. However, skilled masseurs are harder to find and they are not particularly cheap. If new parents cannot afford the high prices, the extended family, or a friend, steps in and helps with the binding. Westerners may question whether it is worth the discomfort and effort. Indonesian mothers provide the answer themselves. They emerge from childbirth like butterflies from the chrysalis. Their skin glows, they radiate energy and their bodies look as good as, if not better than, before the birth.

The Art of Bone Knitting
Indonesians rarely rush to the nearest hospital to emerge with broken bones set in plaster. Instead they head for the bone expert. Interestingly, the highest concentration of bone experts in Java comes from Cisarua, a village near Sukabumi, two hours south of Jakarta. Because of their renown and the relative proximity to Jakarta, they are inundated with patients.

Before laying a hand on the patient, many *dukun patah tulang* (as such people are known) concentrate the mind and say a

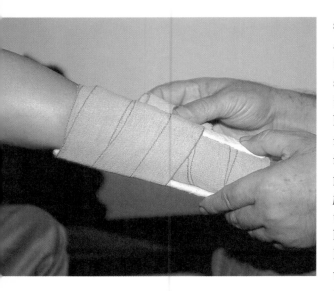

short prayer to consecrate their oil and increase its efficacy. After the massage, patients are often given a bottle of oil with instructions to repeat the treatment at home three times a day, and advised to return when the bottle is empty. Home massage is convenient, for at least one person in most families knows how to massage, or there is a masseur who lives nearby. The routine continues till the bone is healed. These *patah tulang* frequently rectify problems when doctors advise amputation or pronounce injuries incurable. There is no question that *dukun patah tulang* are knowledgeable: they not only possess all the skills of an *urut* expert, but have considerable additional knowledge. While they may not know the scientific or even the Indonesian names for bones, the *patah tulang* is totally familiar with anatomy, physiology and bone structure, muscles and tendons. In this specialist field, it is usual for the trainee to study from books, unlike other massage experts, who learn exclusively by watching and through experience.

The *patah tulang* uses a series of clues to help the diagnosis. Breaks are always accompanied by swelling. If there is no external sign of broken bones, then reddish skin, caused by broken blood vessels, is a good indicator of the affected area. Sometimes the bone expert cannot see a break but can still put the bones back together fairly easily. A bad gash with plenty of blood may appear horrific but joining the bones together is not a real challenge. The difficulty comes only with a combination of broken bones and bleeding that is not visible.

It is important for the massage to begin with the palm about 10 cm (four inches) away from the actual break. By proceeding slowly, the *patah tulang* can feel what kind of break

Above:
Broken bones rarely see a doctor's surgery in Indonesia. Patients automatically consult the patah tulang, *an expert specializing in realigning broken or splintered bones and torn ligaments through massage and use of tiny bamboo splints. These are bound in place with bandages or plasters to keep them in position whilst healing.*

he is dealing with; whether it is jagged, slanted, or a clean break across the bone. Repositioning bones correctly during the early stages of therapy is essential. To relieve the associated pain, the tense, surrounding tendons and muscles are massaged first. The technique is not as simple as it sounds, especially if sharp pieces of bone need to be repositioned. One mistake and an artery can be sliced or a lung pierced. A skilled *patah tulang* is able to recognize when he can help and where his limitations lie. In the latter case, he will refer the patient to the hospital and may in some cases even assist the doctor.

Curative Oils

Oils are used in massage for two reasons, to stop body heat from rising excessively and to make the skin smooth and slippery. Massage professionals often arrive for appointments clutching oils they have prepared themselves. Alternatively they may purchase oils over the counter: Minyak Bulus (Turtle Oil) or Minyak Tawon (Bee Oil; this has nothing to do with bees!). The latter contains nine ingredients: coconut, casuarina, citrus, and terebinthinae oil, which comes from the leaves of a small creeping herb and smells of turpentine; ginger and turmeric roots; garlic, menthol and camphor. An all-rounder, the oil is used to cure headaches, sprains, rheumatism, aching muscles, burns, wounds, ulcers, insect bites and skin infections. For coughs, colds and indigestion, the oil is mixed with warm water and a spoonful of the mixture taken three times a day.

Those who make up their own formulæ tend to stick with three basic oils. One much-used recipe contains 70 per cent yellow coconut oil, 20 per cent musk mallow and 10 per cent lemon grass oil. There are endless combinations and some even include Chinese arak, producing the equivalent of an alcohol rub. People living in remote villages with limited means and choice tend to use less sophisticated versions, such as mixing lime juice, hot water and cooking oil. Vegetable oil, the stock-in-trade of many an *Ibu pijat*, is perfectly adequate but if used straight from the bottle, it can be too thick and tends to create an unpleasant smell when combined with the skin's own odours and body heat.

Of the many oils on sale, a mixture of Minyak Tawon and Lulur Wangi is one of the best. Tawon is warm, providing the healing element, while Lulur gives rough skin the texture of silk. Both white and yellow Lulur are readily available and while Indonesian women favour the yellow variety, the yellow tint it gives the skin is not suitable for Caucasians. Cajuput oil (*minyak kayu putih* from the tree *Melaleuca leucadendra*) is an old reliable standby that cures all manner of aches and pains, flu, fever, headaches, coughs and asthma. Minyak Angin is the same thing with the addition of a few extra ingredients. This is powerful medicine and must be diluted by 70 per cent with basic oil. Families used to keep this oil in the cupboard for emergencies, just as Western mothers stored Friar's Balsam or Vick's.

Genuine experts are loath to pass on their oil-making secrets to anyone, including the immediate family. Apparently, old ladies pray over oils while they are being made. They read the

Above:
Oils are an integral part of the archipelago's health treatments. They are used during massage and taken internally two weeks before giving birth. There are many kinds of oils—either home-made or shop-bought —for rheumatics, relaxation, and general health

Qur'an, invoke the spirits or even solicit help from Satan while they develop their recipes. An unwritten law says these skills cannot be passed down further than three generations. Should they reach a fourth, it is thought too many errors may have crept in to the original treatments, rendering them less effective. If a masseuse feels the next generation has not produced a suitable recipient for the knowledge, it is not passed on either. Sharing knowledge is alien in Indonesian culture, so old women often guard their secrets, forgetting that once they too learnt from an expert.

Massage Moves With the Times
Contrary to what one might imagine, massage is a growing profession. Western practitioners are realizing they have a lot to learn from their Eastern counterparts. Shiatsu, pressure point, reflexology and acupressure are increasingly common subjects in health magazines and at conferences, while the techniques are becoming far more accepted in medical circles and clinics in both Europe and America.

Once, a career in massage had negative connotations and training was only available as part of a beauty course. Today, there are scores of colleges offering qualifications to meet the rising demand. With New Age trends gaining momentum, old-age methods of curing are being re-evaluated. The value of Indonesian massage has at last begun to travel beyond its national borders. As Eastern philosophies continue moving West, these techniques will become more available; people will see for themselves whether or not they work and arrive at their own conclusions.

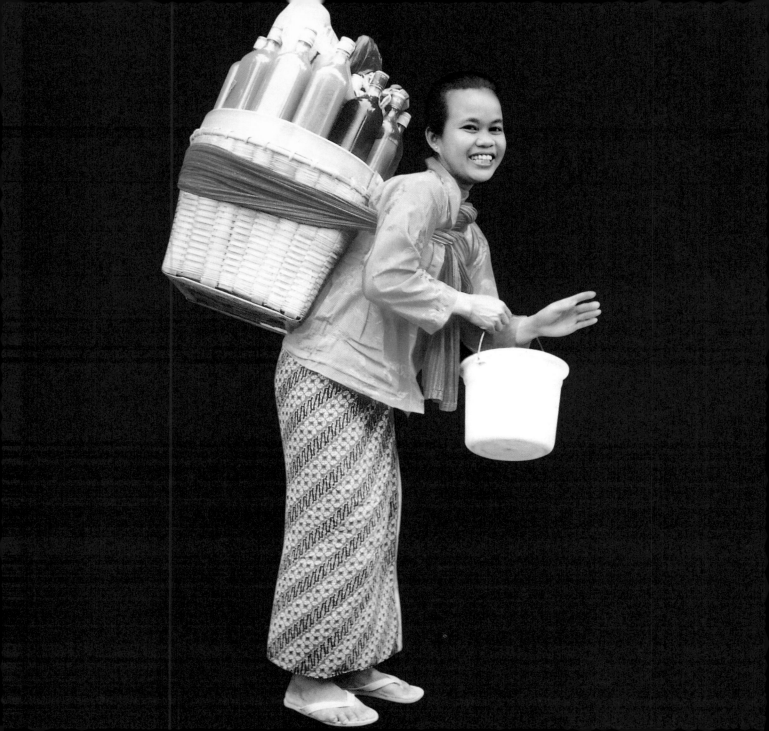

Chapter 5. Healers, Collectors and Gendong

Between the plants in the wild and a satisfied patient, there lies a wealth of knowledge and a network of people, most of whom rarely meet.

Left:
This tiny jamu gendong working in Jakarta routinely carries a load of 22 kg (44 lbs) at the beginning of her daily round.

Between plants in the wild and a satisfied patient, there lies a wealth of knowledge and a network of people, most of whom rarely meet. The healer is inevitably the most revered of this human network, for it is he (or she) who is capable of transforming sickness into health. But he relies, more often than not, on his profound understanding of massage, his extensive experience in and knowledge of herbal medicine, and traditional healing techniques. He will grow his own herbs or buy them from a market or be supplied by pickers working in and around the villages. There is also a second level of supply, namely middlemen or collectors; they obtain stocks from pickers and plantation owners and, in turn, supply the jamu manufacturers located in Java's main cities.

The Healer
There is no such thing as a typical healer in Indonesia because treatments and medicines vary enormously. Healers come from all walks of life and have an extraordinary range of skills. Some discover that they can find a cure to a particular ailment when modern medicine has been unsuccessful; some are born with the gift, while others convert through some personal experience; yet

119

others come to the work through an interest in humanity and the human body; and a small group reverses the trend and expands their modern medical training to include centuries-old, traditional methods. In general, healers tend to rely on a sense of touch, personal experience and an abundance of natural herbs and plants.

As there is no stereotype healer, there is likewise no rule to the method. Their popularity is solely the result of their success. Most will have a thorough knowledge of physiology and anatomy; some may even have come from allopathic medical practice; and many have an untrained gift or have studied under a master. Payment for a healer's skills, as for a masseur's, is arbitrary. A good healer often leaves the fee up to his patient.

Ritual and Healing
Life in Indonesia is steeped in superstition. In Java, for example, numerous rituals have been designed to eliminate negative forces and restore harmony to the environment. Just as Westerners may avoid walking under ladders, regard black cats as unlucky, and salute magpies for good luck, the Javanese have a whole range of their own superstitions. For example, one concerns Javanese giants, beings that are said to represent dirt, disease and disaster: the Javanese will hang a huge mirror opposite the front door, so if a giant opens it, he will see his own reflection and run away in fright!

A *ruwatan* (wiping out) or *supat* (a sin forgiven) is a Javanese exorcism ceremony that mixes pre- and post-Islamic healing practices. A *ruwatan* is not limited to human beings and can be applied to houses or even cars that are giving trouble. The ceremony varies with the problem and the region where it is performed. For instance, in Sunda (West Java), which is famed for its *wayang* puppet performances (shadow puppet theatre), *dalangs* or puppet masters are often mystics of a very high order who also conduct *ruwatan*.

Whether the *ruwatan* is successful or not is almost irrelevant. If people take this precaution and something bad still happens, they can bear it more easily because they know everything possible was done to prevent it. Herbs and food are included in *ruwatan* because people believe the giant or spirit threatening them will eat the food instead of symbolically 'eating' their child or venting its fury on the house. Having restored peace and harmony with a *ruwatan*, one gives thanks by holding a *selamatan*.

Ruwatan can also be preventive. They are often organized at the outset of a new project that may invite trouble, such as building a new house. Here, the ceremony is designed to prevent arguments from breaking out between owner and builder. It also reminds the construction crew to work carefully to avoid accidents, especially at dangerous stages, like putting on a roof. If owners do not hold a ceremony and someone is injured, they will be blamed for this misfortune, which is why these ceremonies are still part of life in modern Java.

Magic and Medicine

Herbs alone cannot always cure. Sometimes prayer and ritual are the answer, but in cases of persistent illness, people often turn to magic. Healers who work with a combination of medicine and magic to cure or cast curses can be found throughout Indonesia, although the Balinese are the acknowledged experts in this field.

A Dutch Priest turns Healer

Father Lukman, a young Dutch priest who came to Central Java in 1965, found jamu fascinating and began studying it seriously. But it was not until 1972 that he began to practise alternative medicine, which he defines as "healing that has an ancient tradition behind it or has been well proven by experience".

Today, Father Lukman's jamu and diagnostic method are well known. He compares its complexities to water divining. "First I plot the technical or architectural design of the patient. I use a metal ball-point or my pectoral cross to detect vibrations from a patient's body, or more specifically, from the nerves. This pinpoints the problem and enables me to build up a clear picture of his or her health." The technique requires keen sensitivity to body vibrations: "Just as the divining rod or twig vibrates near water, I use total concentration to project my sensitivity towards the human body so I can accurately pick up the vibrations it emits." The priest then translates these vibration levels as a series of figures into a code that enables him to identify the problem—and to prescribe a cure.

Father Lukman says there is no relation between his system and mysticism. "Everyone knows that magnetic fields exist: You can have areas of high or low magnetism, and if an imbalance occurs it can be neutralized."

While many Westerners may be sceptical of such matters, foreigners who have lived in Bali for years do not dismiss any form of magic lightly. Things happen that defy normal explanation: people become ill or are cured for no apparent reason.

Balians, who practice black magic, can plant pins, broken glass or razors in victims, to be pulled out later by white magicians. De-materialization is said to be responsible for this phenomenon: when needles are transformed into energy, they can penetrate anything. Such occurrences have no scientific explanation, although the energy theory attracts many supporters.

Interestingly, Indonesians do not distinguish between black and white magic; they argue the same magic that helps one person usually succeeds at the expense of another. Professor Parangtopo, from the Physics Department at the School of Mathematics and Natural Sciences at the University of Indonesia, acknowledges that while supernatural powers exist, he cannot offer any explanation. Such instances are categorized under Metaphysics, and scientists currently understand less than ten per cent of the subject.

In 1985, the journal *Social Science and Medicine* published a study by Mark Woodward on three contemporary healers in Central Java who were aware of their limitations and referred patients with infectious diseases to orthodox doctors. In terminal cases, they suggested only prayer and meditation. These healers utilized a set of shamanistic beliefs and practices, based on *kesakten*, or power that can be used for good or evil. This power is thought to be very dangerous in the hands of unskilled healers. Nonetheless, healers must possess *kesakten* to overcome evil spirits; thus, they command as much fear as they inspire respect.

"Indonesian culture is built on secrets," reveals one of Indonesia's best known healers. "Sharing knowledge is foreign to most Asians, and to Indonesians in particular. For instance, it's difficult for foreigners to marry Indonesians because if problems arise in a marriage the Indonesians always insist everything is fine. It isn't an issue for me because I can enter my husband's subconsciousness!" This healer further remarked that many people do not have the patience to train for this work as it can take around 30 years to become competent.

With the subject (or his photograph) in front of her, this healer matches the vibrations of her mind with those of the patient. She is then literally on the same wavelength as the patient, and can send vibrations or read his thoughts (relayed through a soft whispering in the ear). The crucial spot is the 'third eye' at the centre of the forehead, she says. The all-powerful instrument is the mind, and because it controls the body, healers believe that many illnesses are created by mental imbalance. In the same way that meditation works by increasing energy and replacing negative feelings, this healer passes positive thoughts on to her patients.

A book by Dr Lawrence LeShan, *How to Meditate*, goes far in explaining the unexplainable. The author defines extra sensory perception (ESP) as a collective phrase to cover telepathy, clairvoyance and precognition, and points to evidence that such paranormal occurences include both spontaneous cases and precise laboratory studies.

Trances, meditation and mysticism, which form an important part of healing in Indonesia, are at once fascinating, impressive and even frightening. Western writings on psychic power

---

Banishing the Blues

Healers are often consulted for mental or emotional illnesses, as well as physical ones. In *Serat Centhini* there are a number of healing remedies for psychological conditions. We read of an antidote for sadness which recommends pressing *gambir putih* (*Uncaria gambieri*) flowers together with *semanggi* leaves (*Hydrocotyle sibthorpioides*) and pouring this mixture over the head. The hair should then be twisted hard before the liquid is poured in the other direction, that is, from the ends of the hair over the face. As this procedure has to be carried out with the eyes open, it must have been uncomfortable. Indeed Widuri, the girl afflicted in *Serat Centhini* is said to have "shouted loudly, had difficulty breathing and moaned miserably" during the cure. Nonetheless it was deemed totally effective, according to the book.

Similarly, a distraught mother managed to treat two lovesick daughters using *sirih* or betel leaves (*Piper betel*) that were inscribed with religious symbols and figures. The leaves were sprayed over the girls and that, apparently, was the end of their broken hearts.

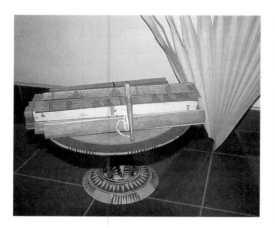

generally concur that it works when practised by highly trained minds, but those less skilled abuse it at their peril or are simply ineffectual, which is what sometimes happens in Indonesia.

Dreams in Healing

In the past, dreams were an integral part of healing. Although the practice is no longer so prevalent, there are still people who firmly believe in dreams and take interpretations very seriously. In many countries, including Indonesia, dreams and other forms of divination have been used—and continue to be used—to determine auspicious times, circumstances, places or even useful ceremonial items. Understanding these and other signs is considered essential to the well being of the population.

Many Indonesians believe that some of the older jamu recipes were received by people while in a trance, or through dreams. It is a subject surrounded by superstition and secrecy, and gaining concrete evidence is difficult, but one fact is certain: dreams, mysticism of one sort or another, and even magic, are an integral part of Indonesian traditional medicine. Highly-educated people in Indonesia accept such hypotheses without question. For example, an extremely forward-thinking, modern member of the royal family in Solo revealed that Javanese royalty acquired much of its knowledge through dreams. She illustrated her point with the story of a young girl from the neighbouring palace who had received jamu formulæ in dreams and founded a large and successful herbal medicine company. "There is no other expla-nation—they came from dreams," she affirmed and made it clear there would be no further discussion or questions on a subject that—in her mind at least—was clearly beyond dispute.

Above:
The traditional tools
for writing on Balinese
lontar *leaves.*

Philosophy Behind the Healing

Indonesians believe that punishment can descend in the form of illness when a vow remains unfulfilled or a taboo is broken. People are also at risk if they commit a sacrilegious act against the guardian spirit of a sacred or haunted place. Not taking good care of sacred possessions, such as family heirlooms, or a curse by an elder are other sources of illness. Finally, black magic can wreak havoc with health unless it is properly handled.

The island of Bali gives us a glimpse of the vibrant society of ancient Hindu Java and the traditions of animist Bali. In the latter, people relied on a combination of belief, prayer, ritual, magic and herbal medicine to solve their health problems. But while herbal remedies like jamu could treat many illnesses, sometimes these alone could not heal, but must be combined with spiritual backup. Without the appropriate ritual, a victim could not recover.

In preventing disturbances from an evil spirit, people believe the answer lies in pictures or writing in Arabic, Balinese or Javanese script. Such antidotes are normally hung on the upper part of a doorway or in places that are thought to be haunted. Many Balinese healers either go into a self-induced trance to speak on behalf of dead ancestors, or put their patients into a state of trance. They then pinpoint the cause of a particular sickness or difficulty with remarkable accuracy. These healers tend to specialize in one particular field: there are herbalists, midwives, pædiatricians, and soothsayers as well as bone and stomach ache experts. Patients, including Westerners, who have experienced Balinese healing will openly attest to the success of their methods.

The Mystical Side of Jamu

Dutch-born Laurentia was only seven or eight years old when she started to see and hear things. During World War II, a presentiment made her refuse to enter an air raid shelter which, minutes later, was hit, leaving a handful of survivors. Her premonition had saved her life.

In her late teens, Laurentia realized her gift was increasing each day. It was then she encountered Madame Hebbelard, a famous healer who used Dutch herbs and also had a sixth sense. The visit sparked off Laurentia's interest in herbalism and she decided to learn more about homeopathy.

When she married, she came to live in Indonesia and began to study herbs seriously. Nyonya Lauren, as she is now known, travelled all over the archipelago, learning and building up her extensive knowledge of herbal practices. On a visit to Ambon, she and her husband witnessed a paralysed old man being repeatedly beaten with stout branches. It transpired this was a local cure: the beatings stimulate blood circulation, warm the skin and open the pores to allow fine powder from flower stamens to stick to the skin and enter the body through the pores, thus starting the healing process. By the end of the week the patient slowly began to move again.

Nyonya Lauren's approach is holistic. She studies the patient's aura in order to make a diagnosis. "You'll notice I always sit with the light behind me, so I can see someone's aura clearly," she says. Once the basic information has been assimilated, Nyonya Lauren works by moving her hands slowly in front of her, looking to see where the aura enters the body. If it goes into the heart and out again, Nyonya Lauren examines that area in detail to check out the problem. The final stage is the divining and prescribing of jamu.

"The aura is a magnetic field around the body comprising a mass of different colours." As she spoke Nyonya Lauren pushed a Polaroid snap of what appeared to be an abstract painting across the desk. "That is a photograph of an aura," she said. It was a mass of reds, yellows and purples, each colour running haphazardly into the next.

"Green on the right side of the body means a bladder problem," she diagnosed, "Yellow indicates the kidneys. Lots of red shows the problem is emotional. Most children have auras composed entirely of soft colours." Over the years, she says she has received many jamu recipes through meditation.

To illustrate her point, Nyonya Lauren cited the case of a cancer patient who showed no improvement after taking the usual medicines. "I got fed up with it," Nyonya Lauren admits, "but I felt there had to be an answer somewhere. I began to meditate intensely and was so at one with her I could feel her pain. Using this technique I received the jamu formula, the types of herbs and the quantities. To my joy, the treatment was successful. You always have to look inside yourself to find the solution—it's an inner feeling." Originally Nyonya Lauren took her formulæ from books, but nowadays she creates special mixtures herself from these "inner feelings". She maintains we all possess such an inner power, we just don't use it.

There are numerous ceremonies designed to wipe out a potential threat, a real threat or to expiate a wrong. Designed for every level of society, and portrayed in symbolic terms similar to the Christian use of parables, they usually involve purification of some nature. For example, the central character in a story could take the form of a vicious animal, a vengeful god or more often a wicked giant, all of which were terrifying to people who had few means of combating epidemics or understanding the root cause of a disease.

The Collector

Before a healer or a jamu-maker can diagnose an illness, make a jamu, or recommend a course of action, they must be supplied with the raw materials of their trade. The rural pickers, often family members of a healer with knowledge of traditional medicine, fill this gap. They are rarely seen because they roam the countryside around their villages, gathering the leaves and plants that are so familiar to them. Some collectors grow medicinal plants and shrubs themselves, but sourcing the raw materials for jamu is usually a more casual, haphazard process.

Good pickers know every plant in their neighbourhood and identify them easily. But even experts make mistakes. This can occur when different varieties of the same plant grow together; pickers are not always able to distinguish between leaves that are suitable for making jamu, and those that are not. Thus, a jamu manufacturer might receive an inappropriate plant species from collectors, which results in exhaustive sorting and unavoidable wastage. To reduce this kind of error and ensure regular supplies, some manufacturers leave out the middleman-collector entirely

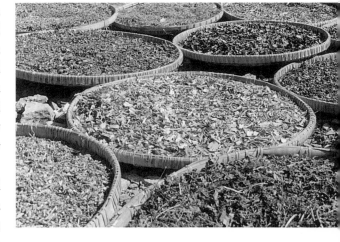

Above:
The rural picker is a key component in the jamu making chain. He may supply his herbs dried, as here, or in raw form.

Curing by Correspondence

Father Lukman, a Dutch priest who combines healing souls with helping the physically sick through his own personal herbal medicine system, has a pragmatic approach to life and his work (see page 121). "I remember one patient with rheumatoid arthritis who was given up as a hopeless case by the doctors," he says. "He tried Dutch jamu which didn't work, then came to me." Father Lukman prescribed some jamu and sent him on his way. A short while later he received a letter from the patient in Holland requesting a repeat order. He wrote: "Please send more of the jamu quickly, I am starting to walk again." "His doctors were dumbfounded," says Father Lukman. "They couldn't believe it. This is why I always invite the medical profession to my practice to see for themselves."

Another patient that Father Lukman treated was a young pregnant mother who, instead of gaining weight, was losing it rapidly through continuous vomiting. Both her own doctor and he agreed she must weigh 50 kg (110 lbs) prior to delivery. He managed to find a formula that arrested the vomiting and encouraged her body to put on weight. Just as she topped the scales at 50 kg, she delivered a healthy child.

All Father Lukman's jamu is registered with the Department of Health and has been subjected to their tests. It is "totally free of chemicals, 100 per cent natural and hygienic". He regrets, however, that much of his jamu cannot be scientifically proven as the components are not known to Western science—a problem shared by many of the country's leading healers.

and buy direct from the villages. They also help small suppliers by investing capital in their business. Another option is distributing seeds and rhizomes to villagers for planting. When leaves, roots and barks are ready for harvesting, the manufacturer buys them back on an exclusive basis.

In recent years, skilled pickers have become increasingly rare. Youngsters do not want this kind of work and the ability to distinguish the various medicinal plants is gradually being lost. The answer may lie in organized cultivation or using specialist commercial growers, but these options have yet to be implemented on any large scale. As the system works currently, the collector's leaves, roots and herbs are mainly sold in the markets and small shops, or go to a middleman who is also confusingly known as the collector. In some cases it is the initial collector who dries his produce, especially when quantities are small, and sells on these dried products to the middleman collector. In other cases it is the middleman who undertakes the drying of jamu ingredients before selling these to the jamu makers.

Such people work long hours. In many areas, the working week of a herbal wholesaler comprises seven days. Their shops often stay open six days a week, while some wholesalers travel to collect fresh raw materials on Sundays.

The collectors are experts on quality—it is in their own interest to ensure that the raw materials accepted will, in turn, be of the quality required for jamu manufacture. Raw materials are usually picked during the dry summer months—May to September—but since factories usually require stocks on a monthly basis, storage is also a consideration. Most herbs are pre-dried and can be kept in sacks for months or even a year.

Most jamu companies purchase raw materials from a mixture of individual and medium-sized growers, or a large collector who can guarantee bulk supplies. Air Mancur, for instance, employ their own collector to source raw materials directly from the villages. Others compromise by buying a small piece of land on which to grow plants that are rare or in short supply, and then buy the remainder outside. For even if they own a plantation, it is almost impossible for factories to grow the diverse range of ingredients they need cost effectively.

The Jamu Gendong

Without doubt, Central Java is the acknowledged home of Indonesian jamu and jamu sellers—*jamu gendong*. Indeed, most jamu sellers or their families originally hailed from the Solo or Yogyakarta area, even though they work all over the country nowadays. Owing to the palace influence, women from this region are said to be highly skilled in making herbal medicine and beauty preparations. Although jamu is almost exclusively the province of women, a small number of men also sell herbal tonics on the streets. Their recipes are restricted to those for general health as a discussion of female problems between a male seller and a female client would be embarrassing.

The *jamu gendong*, who makes her jamu and sells it directly to the customer, is a familiar sight on the streets of Indonesia. It is she, more than anyone else, who brings jamu to the consumer. She sets out early in the morning armed with the tools of her trade: a pail, two glasses and a large basket of bottles of ready-to-drink jamu tied on her back with a long strip of batik. When the bottles are full in the morning, she often carries well over 20 kg

Magical Powers

Even the most educated Indonesians have a healthy respect for the paranormal. Alan, a lecturer in Engineering at Ambon University, says he is usually somewhat sceptical about such matters—but has witnessed a "curse" and cure in his home town countless times.

A river runs in front of the family house in Ambon where locals are welcome to bathe. But if an outsider decides to swim there, he is guaranteed to leave the water with a swollen face and nasty rash covering his body. It has all the makings of a black magic curse.

However, when Alan's great grandfather administers an antidote that looks to be no more than a glass of water, the culprit is cured immediately. Doctors, on the other hand, are baffled by the condition. The antidote is a secret, but Alan says it will pass to the most senior member of the family when his great grandfather dies. "The curse must be pretty strong," says our cynical friend, "Otherwise doctors would be able to deal with it. In these circumstances, a healer must be very powerful to handle such a situation, otherwise the black magic can have a boomerang effect."

(44 lbs). The pail is filled with water for rinsing her dirty glasses and contains a slice of lime to remove the lingering smell of jamu. She walks from door to door selling the freshly made herbal tonics and medicines for which her country is famous.

By tradition, an even number of bottles in a jamu seller's basket means she is married; an odd number shows she is still single. The older, heavy glass bottles are highly prized because they are no longer available. They are passed from one seller to another and are now rarely seen outside the villages of Central Java. The modern alternative is a square Johnny Walker bottle or a plastic mineral water bottle; the latter is frowned upon by purists as it is impossible to sterilize them with boiling water.

On her daily rounds, the *jamu gendong* usually carries four or five popular jamu that maintain or improve health and strength. These jamu are always preventative, rather than curative; she may also have special orders for expensive recipes that are not part of normal stock. *Gendong* also carry factory-made powders for more serious complaints, as well as honey and raw eggs to mask foul taste or to increase the effectiveness of certain jamu.

The itinerant sellers are always well groomed: a smart appearance is good for business. They still wear the elegant full Javanese dress, comprising a tightly-fitting, batik sarong skirt and blouse or *kebaya*. However, they are definitely a dying breed. The older generation often fell into the job because they had littler, or no, schooling, and jamu was a last resort. For their children, who have the benefit of some education, life as a vendor is hardly an option. This, coupled with the fact that commercially produced jamu is now widely available, means the future of this unique profession is not certain.

A Tip for Drivers

Taxi drivers worldwide are expert on handing out gratuitous advice and Jakarta is no exception. The capital's taxi drivers come from every corner of the archipelago and share their culture with enthusiasm.

Pak Agus from Yogyakarta held forth at length and was able to offer the following advice: "Jakarta's horrendous traffic jams mean we drivers suffer from above average stress—it's either headaches, backache or simply fatigue." To keep himself going, Pak Agus swears by a special salad.

"My wife prepares finely sliced *kencur* leaves," he related. "One green chilli, garlic, a little ginger, brown Javanese sugar and salt. I eat it nearly every day. It's served on rice and tastes delicious."

Jamu for Diabetes

The story of Podosalametee—a jamu formulated by Dr Raden Mas Abdulkadir, a member of a high ranking family in Central Java—began in the late 1800s. Dr Abdulkadir had a reputation for being headstrong and rebellious, but he was a fine doctor and travelled widely for the Dutch Government Medical Corps, marrying a much younger woman who accompanied him on his career postings. Through his work Dr Abdulkadir was exposed to a wide variety of plants, patients and diseases. He had ample opportunity to explore herbal alternatives and when Western medicine failed he never hesitated to prescribe traditional treatment. Highly respected, his combination of orthodox and herbal medicine produced results.

These factors enabled Dr Abdulkadir to develop a cure for diabetes from *daun sambiloto* (leaves of the jujube tree; *Andrographis paniculata*), *biji lamtoro* (seeds of Chinese petay tree; *Leucaena glauca*), *bubukan pule* (ground *pulai* wood; *Alstonia scholaris*) and binding materials. He soon found it was equally effective for rheumatism, boils and skin diseases, lowering cholesterol and reducing high blood pressure. He provided the plant and scientific input while his young wife, a herbal medicine expert whose knowledge came from a childhood in the *kraton*, took care of the production.

"Podosalametee", which means to "to save yourself from harm" (in Javanese), may not be an advertising man's dream choice of name, but it was selected with care. Its fame spread as patients and Dutch pharmacies asked for the herbal medicine. Although the Abdulkadirs never advertised and the doctor hadn't any plans to turn Podosalametee into big business, sales steadily increased.

Much of Podosalametee's popularity rests on the fact that it doesn't require patients to follow a strict diet. It can be taken for longer periods than other diabetic medicines without causing side effects. When patients stop taking it, their sugar levels stabilize instead of rocketing up, as often happens with competitive products. Its main purpose is to make organs of the body function normally, so it also contributes to overall health.

Podosalametee is produced in spotless conditions behind the family house and has undergone a series of rigid clinical trials. However, the family has to date resisted overtures by the Department of Health, who would like to increase output because it would mean moving from cottage industry to full scale factory production. Currently, around 5,000 packets of these tiny pills are sold each month.

"We give away as much again in free samples," the doctor's daughter, Nyonya Harjono, admits. "If someone is recommended to us by a friend and arrives with an empty packet, we automatically give them five more without charging a single rupiah—rich or poor—it doesn't matter, our policy is the same."

However, the final words belong to the man who formulated Podosalametee. Dr Abdulkadir always believed in "not much money but masses of friends", and that's the way this cottage industry wishes to remain.

A Cottage Industry

Most *jamu gendong* sell alone. The production of jamu, on the other hand, is something which often involves the entire family. The tedious yet extremely important task of grinding herbs is energy-sapping and requires stamina. In some households, the menfolk help out with the heavy work. The business can thus afford the opportunity for all members of the family to work productively together. The income generated by a skilled *gendong* with a large number of customers can make a substantial economic difference to the income of a small Indonesian household.

Once, a *jamu gendong* would grow many of her own herbs, but nowadays these self-supplying herbalists are rare, and the local markets provide her apothecary. A true *jamu gendong* looks for the freshest ingredients and bargains the seller down to her price. She prepares the raw materials at home by grinding them with a *gandik*, the Indonesian equivalent of a pestle, until they are reduced to a paste. Some jamu sellers do the first grinding the evening before, ready to make jamu early the next morning. Others do all the grinding and making each morning before setting off on their rounds. Reputable jamu sellers use only boiled water to ensure their jamu is free of impurities. Roots and leaves are not generally boiled, but Javanese sugar is bought in cake form and boiled to a liquid before being added to the mixture.

Major companies like Martina Berto and Sido Muncul invest heavily in the *jamu gendong* because these companies sell large quantities of powdered jamu. Each Lebaran (the festival marking the end of the Muslim fasting month) sees a steady stream of buses, sponsored by the two organizations, fetching sellers home

A Taste of Tradition

Ibu Nur of Yogyakarta, now fifty-five years old, was widowed many years ago. Having to single-handedly support five young sons made her turn to life as a *jamu gendong* in an effort to try and scrape together a living for the family. Her boys remember having to go without food when it rained and the jamu didn't sell. Sometimes, when there was no rice to cook, they would survive on Indonesian porridge instead.

"We went to school barefoot because there was no money for shoes," recalls one of Ibu Nur's sons. "And we studied by oil lamps. But we accepted what we had and didn't complain."

When they went to university, the boys helped the family business by ferrying bottles of jamu to and from campus to sell. Their mother was by then well-known for the quality and taste of her jamu, and lecturers placed regular orders. It may be the case that successful children often look down on parents of humble origin, but Ibu Nur's sons were different, and were eager to set the record straight.

"We are not ashamed that our mother is a jamu seller," they insist. "If it were not for her hard work, we wouldn't have achieved anything." For this family, jamu profits tipped the scales and they not only survived difficult times, but they are now also moderately well-off.

Ibu Nur's sons, now all married with families of their own, have repeatedly asked their mother to retire and take life easy. She has steadfastly refused, claiming that "I'll be bored and become fat and old if I don't have the daily exercise and social contact I enjoy through my work."

Ibu Nur says she concentrates on jamu for maintaining health. Her recipes include Beras Kencur and Kunir Asem, Galian for slimming, Enkoo for increasing appetite, a form of cough mixture, and Cabe Puyang for tiredness, or when the body temperature swings between perspiring and shivering.

But why does Ibu Nur still cart jamu around in heavy, old-fashioned glass bottles when sellers in Jakarta use old Johnny Walker or plastic bottles? She explains: "Plastic smells and affects the jamu's taste. What's more it's unhygienic—how do you clean bottles properly if you can't use boiling water?"

The Health Ministry's efforts to improve standards of cleanliness are obviously having an effect. For similar reasons, *jamu gendong* refuse to use electric mixers, as they say the smell from previous mixtures lingers in the bowl and is very difficult to remove.

What about retirement for Ibu Nur? "I cope quite well with eight bottles, the glasses and my bucket," she retorts. "That bucket is more than 20 years old and it's still going strong." In the picture below, she and her aunt (on left) are setting off on their morning round.

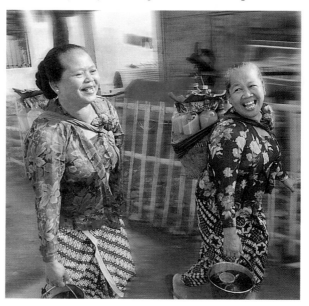

Below:
A famous *jamu*
gendong *statue,*
situated in Wonogiri,
Central Java, often
called the home
of jamu.

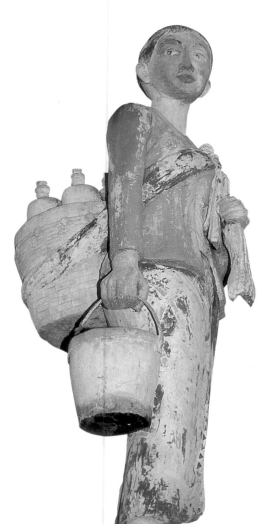

to their families in Sukoharjo and Cirebon. The companies also provide training courses, promotions and competitions throughout the year. Many of these women cannot read and write, but they can make curing jamu, and even experts, such as pharmacist Professor Dr Sidik of Universitas Padjadjaran in Bandung, are studying their methods. The professor first became interested when he met a patient who had been successfully treated by a *jamu gendong* for a liver problem with jamu made from *temu lawak* and red sugar. Extensive clinical trials produced impressive results. Professor Sidik added turmeric to further improve the formula and it has now gone into production under the name of Cursil.

The *jamu gendong* may be a one-woman enterprise, but she provides us with a very accurate picture of Indonesia's herbal medicine in its original form. Her knowledge has hardly changed as it has passed from generation to generation, making her the custodian of today's authentic jamu formulæ. Collectively, *jamu gendong* form the largest group of jamu sellers in Indonesia, numbering some 80,000. The medium- and large-scale factories that emerged in the 19th and 20th centuries owe their existence to the humble *gendong* who laid the foundations of service, trust and reliability, which grew with their makers. These were the people who turned one-woman businesses into cottage industries, some of which have emerged as giants of Indonesia's modern jamu industry.

Cooperation between Gendong
Over the years, cooperatives in Indonesia have embraced a wide range of activities and small commercial ventures, which range

Muntilan's Chinese Jamu Seller

Strangely enough, many Indonesian Chinese are experts on jamu. Chinese have lived in Indonesia for several generations, and some of the earliest Chinese traders who came to Java stayed and married local girls. Generally Chinese Indonesians such as Ibu Kwik Siok Ming's family are totally accepted by villagers who do not make any distinction. Seventy-four-year-old Ibu Ming runs a busy store in Muntilan, a small town close to Yogyakarta. She has run the shop since 1950, assisted for the past 20 years by her daughter-in-law, a local Muntilan girl.

Ibu Ming says that she never needs to go to the doctor because she takes Jamu Cabe Puyang every day. She believes good health is a matter of mental discipline. "If you don't think about the evil of your fellow man," she says wisely. "You have peace of mind and that's important for good health."

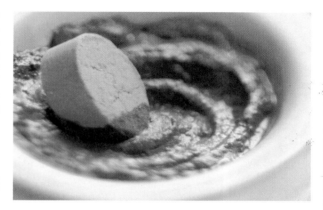

Wrapping medicine is an art all its own here. The jamu is prepared in battered, old, tin mugs. Water and herbs are mixed together and sieved. More herbs are added before a second sieving takes place, then the sediment is squeezed and washed out of the mug into the sieve. The end product is transferred to a small plastic bag which is carefully knotted. This plastic bag is packed into a banana leaf and finally the whole thing is wrapped in a sheet of scrap pad and secured with a rubber band. Only then does money change hands—and the customer leave with a purchase.

"There is no fixed price here, anyone who comes will be helped because many of our customers are poor. I never mention price." Ibu Ming learnt how to make 'instant' Javanese jamu from her mother and grandmother. She buys other jamu in packets and makes it up adding her own spices where necessary. Even the camphor-based compress is bought in packs but prepared in the shop.

"My ingredients and jamu come from everywhere," explains Ibu Ming. "We have many herbs from India such as *Artemisia*

absinthium or wormwood flower buds, but I can also buy these from Solo. *Masoyi* (*Cryptocarya massoy*) is also Indian and is used to make curry gravy and in Cabe Lempuyang. The Indian fruit, *jenitri* (*Elæocarpus ganitrus*), tightens the vagina. *Legi* (*Glycyrrhiza glabra*) is Chinese and very sweet."

In keeping with the best jamu shops, Ibu Ming offers advice on complaints, corrects customers if she considers there is a better way of dealing with a problem, and mixes up her own potions for instant consumption. Tiredness, a girl's first menstruation, loss of appetite, fever in a baby, high blood pressure, cough remedy and a deterrent for a child who still wanted to be breastfed at three, were just some of the challenges Ibu Ming faced in an hour's work. She also sold to a *gendong* with a basket full of jamu. The woman purchased some packets of jamu from Ibu Ming because "it suits my regulars", she said.

"For headaches," Ibu Ming announces, "we buy powder from Semarang and make up the *pilis* here by adding hot water." It had a wonderful smell of cloves, and when the author tried this cure, her *pilis* was so effective that 15 minutes after application, her headache had disappeared.

from the production of handicrafts, batik, ceramic and furniture to taxis, milk, tempe and, inevitably, jamu. Although these are admittedly small fry compared with their bigger siblings, the jamu cooperatives are lively and productive. They also enjoy strong support from the Ministry of Health, which runs courses to improve the jamu sellers' skills and standards of cleanliness and monitors the results.

Jamu gendong often join a cooperative in their area. For example, there are four in the capital and many more in the jamu-making areas of Central Java. The advantages of such an arrangement are considerable for members working in Jakarta who often buy dried ingredients from their own villages, which guarantees fresh materials at lower prices. Division of labour means that home-staying members are able to concentrate on jamu making and continue the role of childcare, while others—even those who are mothers—go out selling for a couple of hours each day.

The life of a *jamu gendong* is not an easy one. The work is hard, the hours are long, and the rewards are not great. Besides making effective jamu, the *jamu gendong* needs to concentrate to a certain extent on her own appearance. She needs to look good, for who will buy her jamu if she is not a walking advertisement for her products? Furthermore, she needs to keep her regular customers happy, but also concentrate at the same time on increasing the amount of jamu she sells. If a *jamu gendong* can successfully balance this equation, with careful management her earnings should be able to support a family of five or more.

In Search of a Cure for Cancer

Professor Dr Asmino, an eminent radiologist, was raised and educated in East Java. During the five years that he worked in the Radiology Department of Universitas Indonesia, where he graduated, he also completed a three-year post-graduate radiology course in the US. In 1968 he was appointed Professor of Radiology at Surabaya's highly respected Universitas Airlangga. Until his death, the doctor was consultant to a cancer clinic and frequently lectured at international medical conferences.

As with many Indonesians, Dr Asmino was brought up on jamu and recalled that his mother knew exactly what to do when one of the 14-strong family was sick. Thus, he was familiar with *sogo telik* (*Abrus precatorius*; bead plant), used for general health or asthma; *legundi* leaves (*Vitex trifolia*; Indian privet) for kidney stones; *kenikir* (*Cosmos caudatus*, a kind of gardenia), *luntas* leaves (*Pluchea indica*) or cloves, whose oils have a drying effect. His favourite remedy was a herbal wrap for cold and fatigue, made from a mixture of pounded grated ginger and *gandapura* oil (Wintergreen oil; *Gaultheria procumbens*).

In September 1988, Dr Asmino found he could pass only small amounts of urine and often made three trips to the bathroom at night. Diagnosed with advanced prostate cancer, he selected minimal surgery over radiation or chemotherapy, which could interfere with his immune system. He also chose alternative medicine though he was acutely aware that jamu's healing powers and dosage required detailed research. Close friends also recommended consultation with Haji Hani Ahmad, better known as Haji Lele, a 51-year-old healer with a high success rate in helping terminal patients. His treatment included pinching the toes and taking two spoons of natural honey every morning. Dr Asmino's urine flow improved dramatically and he passed a white custard-like jelly. Then, in March 1992, the doctor's sense of taste disappeared. He now replaced his daily vitamin C intake with multi-vitamins. Finally, he also took Islamic medicine, accompanied by a ceremony involving the slaughter of three sheep. His tastebuds were re-activated.

Throughout his illness, Dr Asmino examined countless alternatives, demonstrating an open mind and an indomitable spirit. One such option was a famous Indonesian cancer cure: parasite tea, obtained from tea plantations in the Puncak mountains outside Jakarta. Later, he used mango parasite instead, a cheaper substitute. Mistletoe leaves also proved effective. The professor later read, the viscotoxin in mistletoe kills the tumour while lectin strengthens the immune system. In Europe this cure is so popular that extract of mistletoe, Eurixor, is available from pharmacies. Since early 1991, he began taking two to four raw *daun dewa* leaves (leaf of divinity; *Gynura procumbens* var. *Macrophylla*) daily. Known in Java as *sambung nyawa* ("prolonging the soul or life"), the leaves are often also prescribed for removing warts, allergies, itching, stomach complaints, wounds, high blood pressure, cholesterol, and even bee stings. The healing element is saponin in the leaves.

Dr Asmino was a consultant to Yayasan Wisnuwardhana, a charity that treats cancer patients using Hyoko mushrooms and shark cartilage. "Finally I am so convinced of the therapeutic qualities of these two treatments that I have stopped looking for other cancer cures," he said. "Using these, I feel happy, healthy, like a fish in water."

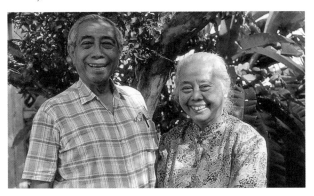

Jamu Maker to the Stars

The warmth and friendliness of Pak Suryo Ing Alogo are, upon meeting him, immediately apparent. A spiritual strength seems to radiate from the man, making one aware of his intelligence and the power of his personality.

Pak Suryo is a well-known maker of traditional Indonesian remedies. Just 15 years ago, he was equally famous as one of Indonesia's leading film producers. The events which changed his life began the morning he successfully negotiated the contract for a new film. This achievement should have been cause for celebration; however, by that evening, his euphoria had strangely disappeared and Pak Suryo was in turmoil. He had received a strong and unusual message, which he believed came from God.

Pak Suryo belonged to a non-political spiritual group for years and was used to listening out for messages. He explains: "The purpose of the spiritual group was for members to communicate directly with God without an intermediary." Pak Suryo learned to accept that when he prayed for guidance and none was forthcoming, it was God's way of saying that whatever he sought was not his destiny at that time. However, now, he was receiving a message, and it was urging him to help people by making jamu. After much thought, he decided to ignore the message and he continued to make films until, suddenly, he became ill. Despite the symptoms, doctors were unable to diagnose his sickness, let alone cure it. His condition deteriorated, and in total despair, Pak Suryo turned, once again, to God.

"I said to God: take my life, I am completely in your hands. Instantly I felt the pressure to become a jamu expert returning; it was stronger than ever." This time he vowed he would follow the instruction. "The following morning, I awoke to find the symptoms had completely disappeared," he exclaimed. "Everything felt normal again." Puzzled doctors checked Pak Suryo repeatedly and pronounced him 100 per cent fit. He was discharged, and began the preparation to start making jamu while still continuing his film career.

To his amazement, Pak Suryo found once he began, research was unnecessary—knowledge simply appeared. Whatever he needed to know about roots, plants, herbs and formulæ was instantly available in his head. Quantities presented themselves to him as he strove to follow God's will. He swears his only contribution was to learn Latin to identify the scientific names of jamu ingredients, and even that came easily to him. He had only to read a book once and he would remember it by heart. There was no doubt in Pak Suryo's mind—he had been chosen as an instrument of God.

Word spread quickly and Pak Suryo's practice grew. He discovered he could treat many illnesses, including those which defeated orthodox medicine. To his surprise, Pak Suryo realized he could also tell when a patient was the victim of black magic. "Of course I never informed them," he said, "because most people simply wouldn't believe me; I just cured them anyway."

Pak Suryo explained that the supernatural is not an everyday occurrence. Usually, he treats more common ailments, such as epilepsy, tuberculosis and diabetes. He is particularly known for his slimming jamu, which is available in three strengths, depending on how fast the patient wishes to lose weight. His list of clients reads like a Who's Who of Indonesia and includes other medical practitioners.

The 40 different recipes Pak Suryo uses are adapted to suit the individual patient. By touching a patient's wrist, he can instantly see the complete picture, because a medical history and analysis flash up in front of him. This ability enables him to provide what is in essence a totally holistic treatment. To the sceptics, Pak Suryo explains his diagnostic method by comparing it to the behaviour of a new-born, which he feels is a clear analogy: both rely on instinct. Pak Suryo is adamant his formulæ come from within, unlike other jamu makers who say their knowledge is received via dreams. Nothing is written down—it's all in his head.

Over the years, Pak Suryo has compared his formulæ with doctors' prescriptions as well as health and beauty recipes from manuscripts in the *kraton* library at Yogyakarta. Surprisingly, he notes, in essence the formulae are usually the same. He thinks there may be some tenuous link for this, as it transpired that Pak Suryo's father was the grandson of Hamengkubuwono V, one of the sultans of Yogyakarta who reigned from 1822–1855.

Pak Suryo may have a gift from God, and he may have cured numerous people, but there have been some patients whom—for some reason—even he cannot help. When asked to elaborate on what actually happened during such situations, he said: "At times like this my mind goes blank. My gift simply doesn't exist any more. It is not even connected with whether or not I like the person—that is irrelevant. I experienced this problem when I saw a patient who was paralysed and couldn't walk. It occurred again when I saw a migraine sufferer. A few days later I tried again with the same result. Shortly afterwards I heard both patients had died. I think this is God's way of protecting me."

The source of Pak Suryo's miraculous healing and jamu recipes may be too much for the cynical Western mind to accept. However, the fact still remains that Pak Suryo was a highly respected, successful film maker before his career in jamu was suddenly thrust upon him. He uses traditional formulæ which work, and hundreds of people from both the East and West will attest to the efficacy of his cures.

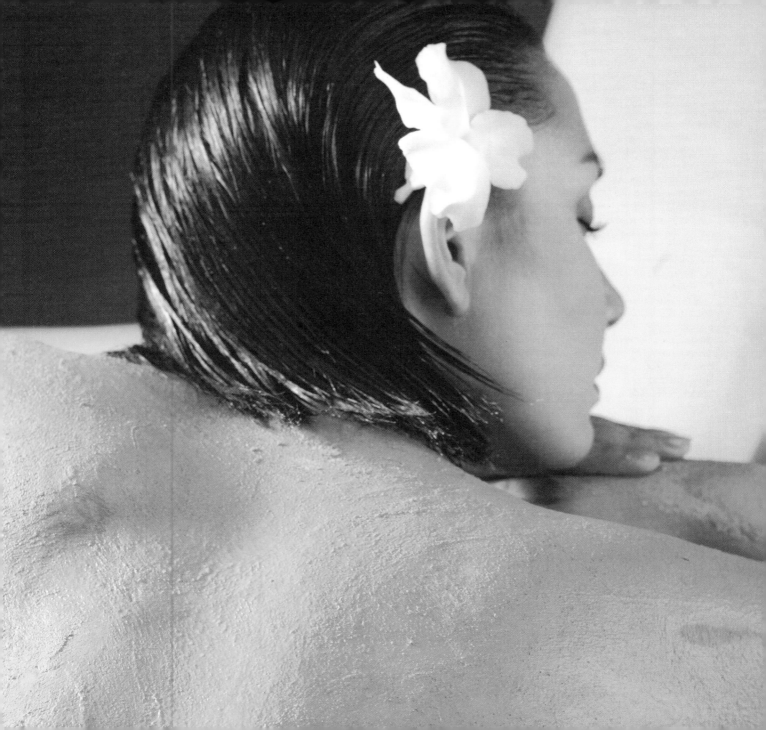

Chapter 6. Beauty from Within

In essence, beauty care in Indonesia is a total beauty system for mind and body: to Indonesians, traditional medicine and beauty products are an integral part of the same programme.

Left:
Beauty in Indonesia is seen as internal and external. Jamu takes care of internal beauty ensuring a woman is in perfect health to give her glowing skin, good figure and beautiful hair whilst massage, skincare and cosmetics provide a result of breathtaking beauty.

Looking good is a way of life for every Indonesian woman. Traditional beauty secrets are taught alongside the philosophy that a woman is responsible for maintaining her own health and beauty. The art of total beauty, particularly hair care, is recorded in temple reliefs from the 9th to 17th centuries, but nobody had access to these secret recipes without royal permission. Only a select few knew exactly which ingredients fashioned the exotic potions of the *kraton*.

Although the palaces do not wield the same influence as in the past, their power within their region still remains strong. Life behind the *kraton* walls goes on as before, and ordinary people still try to emulate court customs. Thus, much traditional beauty care is intact. Within the palaces, lessons in health and beauty began in childhood. A Javanese princess or lady of rank received a daily massage and *lulur* (an abrasive herbal paste) rub, made from rice, pulverized bark and flowers. This paste leaves the skin soft, clean, smooth and gives Asian skin a golden glow. In later years, it helps to slow the wrinkling and ageing process. At court, *lulur* was followed by a herbal bath. Then came an intricate hairstyle and makeup session, and finally the selection of clothing and jewellery. Before bed a female courtier stood over a brazier for 15 minutes while a rich, fragrant smoke perfumed her body in readiness for the royal bedchamber.

Palace manuscripts explain that outer beauty is achieved with an almost unlimited array of herbal skin creams and lotions. Inner beauty is much more demanding as it requires both mental and physical effort. It involves drinking jamu and following a tough regime of fasting and introspection.

In essence, beauty care in Indonesia is a total beauty system for mind and body: to Indonesians, traditional medicine and beauty products are an integral part of the same programme. Originally the mixtures were ostensibly designed for health and beauty, but their underlying purpose was to preserve family unity (it was believed that if the woman was beautiful and took care of herself, the man would not stray!).

Jamu Throughout a Woman's Life Cycle

Javanese women are introduced to jamu right from birth, but the first real lesson comes when a girl begins menstruating. To give their blessing, her female relatives and friends sprinkle her with perfumed water. They are then served with special food. The girl is given Jamu Gadis (virgin jamu). This is made with a little earth she picks up from the garden with three fingers and adds to the ingredients, which are then steamed. The ceremony symbolizes the girl's entry into womanhood, her physical and spiritual fertility, future resilience to and recovery from the rigours of menstruation and childbirth, and her eternal love for family and friends.

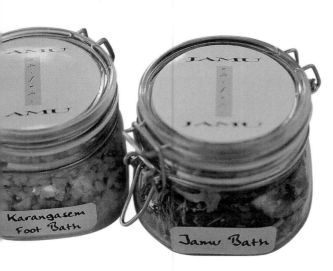

Above:
Products from Jamu-Jamu, a company that runs spas in Bali.

Her next serious encounter with jamu is when she prepares for her wedding. At one time a bride-to-be was confined to her bedroom 40 days before the event, fed a carefully balanced diet, and given *lulur* daily, because she was required to be her most beautiful on her wedding day. Traditionally, a new bride was judged by her husband and the community on her herbal medicine skills and ability to care for her family. Jamu-making was thus essential and also determined how well she kept her looks and her husband. Even now, the day before the wedding, the woman takes a perfumed steam bath so that she will have a fresh and cool body, velvety skin and sweet breath. As a final touch, she drinks a draught of a special jamu, concocted to heighten desire. These days, this is often Jamu Kamajaya Kamaratih, made by Mustika Ratu and named after a famous loving couple in the shadow puppet theatre.

Throughout her life, jamu is a woman's support system: it guarantees a harmonious home life and is the answer to physical problems. There is Jamu Langsing, which removes excess fats and liquids; Galian Singset, which tones the body and tightens muscles; and Jamu Parem, which helps the body stay sexily curvy if a woman becomes too thin. For exhaustion there are potions such as Kolasom, a tonic wine. The choice of jamu is endless. Mustika Ratu's Jamu Sedet Saliro, for example, contains *jati belanda* leaves (bastard cedar) and *bengle* (purple ginger; *Zingiber cassumunar*), both of which are known to keep the female body firm and slim. Jamu Pare Anom, made from *bunga srigading* (flower from the tree of sadness; *Nyctanthes arbor-tristis*), helps a woman stay young, while *botor* (a type of bean; *Psophocarpus tetragonolobus*) is for fine, glowing skin.

Below:
These hard balls are mixed with water to produce a face mask, that refreshes, tightens and tones the skin.

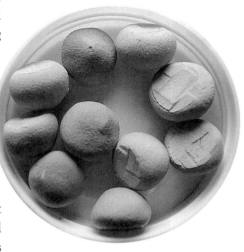

143

Pregnancy, Post-Natal Care and the Later Years

Jamu Hamil Muda (early-pregnancy jamu) will see expectant mothers safely through the first six months of pregnancy. For the remaining weeks, she should switch to Jamu Hamil Tua (late-pregnancy jamu). After birth, maternity jamu, like Jamu Darmi's Galian Luntur, purifies the blood, cleanses the womb and fights off infection during the seven days after delivery. Galian Bersalin then strengthens the womb and helps restore the body to its former shape. If the womb is not properly cleaned, the mother may experience irregular periods and painful, swollen breasts, which indicate impurities still remain. For this, Jamu Luntur or Jamu Nifas is used because it contains a mild abortifacient which thoroughly cleanses the womb. A herbal sit-bath to soothe and restore swollen tissue helps. The mother is also encouraged to do vaginal exercises to strengthen the muscles.

Jamu Darmi's Tapel or Poultice B is another example of an external remedy working together with jamu. The poultice reinforces the work of Jamu Galian Bersalin by tightening the overstretched skin of the stomach from the outside. For slow recovery, fatigue, or headaches and dizziness, a compress made by Air Mancur is effective, as is Jamu Darmi's delightfully named 'Star in Your Eyes', a *pilis* that is applied to the forehead.

Exotic Fragrances

No woman's beauty routine is complete without perfume. Fragrances came mostly from flowers but one of the most popular was musk oil. Courtiers used this oil to make an incense called *dedes*. It even travelled to Europe, where ladies from the Court of Versailles considered it a rival to French perfumes.

In *The History of Jawa*, published in 1817, Sir Stamford Raffles noted that Indonesian ladies loved fragrances such as sandalwood, *gandapura* (musk mallow), *kluangan* (patchouli; *Pogostemon cablin*), orange, *gaharu* (*Aquilaria malaccensis*) and *kelembak* (Java rhubarb) oil. Today, women can enjoy the combination of *kelembak* (*Rheum* sp.), *mangir* (barks used in body scrub creams) and floral essence, which are the ingredients of the popular product called Lulur Sari Bunga. They can also opt for natural oils, made from sandalwood or *akar wangi* (vetiver; *Vetiveria zizanioides*), which smell wonderful on warm skin. Pulverized roots and leaves, such as turmeric, rose myrtle and *temu giring* (a type of ginger), are used in a mixture of *lulur* and mangir, to render the skin smooth, clean and fragrant.

Mustika Ratu makes Jamu Kesepuhan, for those experiencing menopause. It encourages relaxation, improves blood circulation and aids digestion. In old age, other jamu take over: Jamu Pare Anom, a revitalizing formula, delays the ageing process, prevents wrinkles, keeps skin firm, prevents hair from turning white, and reputedly guards against tooth loss. Sari Beras Kencur from Jamu Darmi guards against low blood pressure, certain rheumatic complaints and poor blood circulation.

Lotions, Potions and Cosmetics: A Dazzling Array
Today, few Indonesians make jamu at home because the process takes too long, and the ingredients are often difficult to find. Only the simple practices are still followed, for example left-over tea water (which has mild astringent and antioxidant properties) is put outside overnight for cleansing the face, preventing wrinkles, and rinsing the hair to discourage hair loss. Dandruff

Nyonya Meneer: A Big Name in Beauty

The life of Nyonya Meneer, of the original Nyonya Meneer jamu company, perfectly illustrates how jamu worked to preserve the family unit in the early 1900s. At the age of 16, she became the third wife of a man who had a reputation as a womaniser. The third Nyonya Meneer was exceedingly beautiful and the marriage was set for a fairytale future. However, after a short while, Nyonya Meneer's mother started hearing the old rumours again.

Concerned for her daughter's happiness and learning that Nyonya Meneer was pregnant, her mother decided to take action. To keep the girl healthy, she arrived each morning with home-made jamu. After Nonni was born, Nyonya Meeer's mother switched her daughter to jamu for cleaning the womb and making her muscles contract.

The family moved to Semarang a little later. Nyonya Meneer's mother wrote down her jamu recipes to ensure her daughter's continuing youth and beauty, and packed them into the luggage. Nyonya Meneer began making up the recipes and inevitably, one day, a neighbour arrived whilst she was busy. Enquiring as to its effect, Nyonya Meneer revealed that she drank jamu every day to keep herself young and attractive.

Consequently it wasn't long before Nyonya Meneer had a constant flow of neighbours visiting her on some pretext or other in order to try the jamu. "They asked for bottles to take home," relates Ibu Nonni. "While my mother was happy to make a bit extra, she had no intention of parting with her precious recipes." It was to be the start of a small home-based business.

"Local women soon decided it must be the jamu that was keeping her bold husband at home," Ibu Nonni says. Demand for his wife's herbal medicines increased and she found she had a business on her hands. In 1919, she set up a small factory using a traditional grinding stone to crush and make the jamu. Her selection of jamu constantly changed to match the needs of her neighbour-customers. She would consult her mother's recipe book and prepare what was required.

The original business has now grown into a major group, but the family still uphold their mother's traditional approach. Jamu and cosmetics are designed to complement one another to maximise health and beauty. This is reflected in their brochure which contains over a hundred products divided into separate sections for female, cosmetic and family care herbs; followed by masculine, health promoting and curing herbs.

As one of Indonesia's most celebrated brands of cosmetics and jamu, Nyonya Meneer products are frequently recommended by Western-trained doctors because of their outstanding quality and performance.

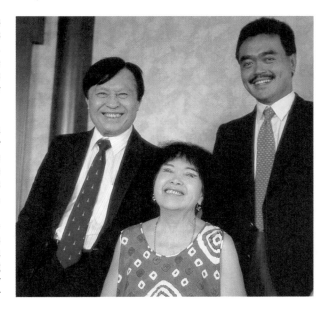

can be treated with pineapple and the scalp can be rubbed with aloe vera to encourage new hair growth. Hence, business has increased for *jamu gendong,* and sales of factory-manufactured jamu are escalating. Although jamu can achieve results on its own, it works more quickly and effectively when combined with complementary beauty products. To this end, some jamu companies have developed an integrated range of jamu, skin care and make-up. Martina Berto is an example.

The company makes a complete range of products using Indonesian herbs as active ingredients. For normal skin, Sari Ayu Cananga, a cleanser made with *kenanga,* prevents dryness and removes any trace of dirt and make-up. A matching toner heals, moisturizes, cleanses pores and restores the skin's natural acid balance. For dry skin, lotions made from fresh essence of Java rose and other ingredients moisturize and soften the skin. Olive cream also guards against dryness. For preventing wrinkles and rejuvenating the skin round the eyes, Mujisat Mata Kejora oil (Miracle Morning Star Eyes) contains a high concentration of natural oils. The Bidari Laut firming face mask, made from bitter *bidara laut* wood, rice starch and honey combined with an oil-based massage cream, completes the range.

For dry skin, Pelembut Wajah (Soft Face) night cream restores moisture balance and keeps skin supple with vitamins A and E. As double insurance, Pelembut Wajah rejuvenating cream reinforces the effect, brightens complexions and improves blood circulation. There is also a quail-egg and honey rejuvenating mask to ensure smooth, strong skin. Oily skin is treated with a range based on fresh lemon essence and a Bidari Laut face mask prepared, again, from *bidara laut* wood and rice starch, but

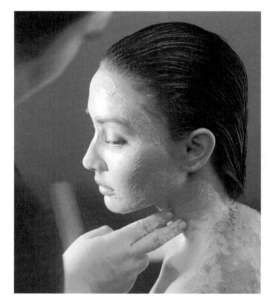

Above:
Lulur wangi *being applied to the skin making it silky smooth to the touch and delicately perfumed.*

Severe Skin Problems

June Coe is married to an engineer who has worked on projects all over the world. As a result, she has coped with a host of different climates and conditions without suffering any ill effects. However, when she moved to Hong Kong some years ago, her hands started causing trouble. The skin became cracked, red, swollen and extremely painful. The doctor diagnosed it as an allergy—and it didn't heal until they moved to another country.

During the eight years the Coes lived in Indonesia, June's hands were periodically sore but the problem disappeared on their return to England. Two years later they were back in Jakarta and the long-forgotten skin complaint reappeared. This time, she decided to try some jamu pills called Kamal, which had been advertised on television and were purportedly made specially for allergies by a company named Borobudur. Kamal worked—her hands were cured in three days.

The instructions on the pack stated: "Very effective for skin diseases such as itch, scabies, skin rash, allergy, itch caused by louse (infested) water etc, and to protect from mosquito bite and so speed up the curing process of wound." The makers emphasize active alkaloid ingredients in their herbs produce excellent results for skin disorders. June's hands did periodically suffer again but a course of Kamal always remedied the problem. June's conclusion?

"If you find the right jamu, it seems to work when other products don't!"

with astringent tamarind pulp included. There are also products to combat skin problems associated with hot, damp tropical climates, such as patchy pigmentation.

These cosmetic products can be used together with suitable jamu. For example, Sari Ayu Jamu Pamor (*pamor* meaning lustre) combines Javanese turmeric and wild ginger, for digestion and skin toning, with *temu giring* (*Curcuma heyneana*) and other herbs, to improve blood circulation and increase vitality. The result is healthy, radiant skin. Although the dosage is ten pills three times a day, it is worth the effort. In addition to the skin products, taking a slimming or rejuvenating jamu at the same time is highly recommended. Jamu Awet Muda (Lasting Youth Jamu), a vitamin E-rich mix of turmeric and black soybean sprouts, promotes the growth of healthy cells and revitalizes the body by improving the digestion and absorption of nutrients.

Not all the problems experienced in the Western world are the same as those in the East, or vice versa. A tropical climate can help beauty care because skin perspires, a natural process that forces impurities out through the pores. Therefore, clogged pores—the bane of city-dwellers in Europe—are rare in Asia, particularly since most people shower twice a day. Climate is also the reason Indonesian women use Bedak Dingin or Cooling Powder for the face. The famous rice powder, mixed with rose water for normal skin, or fresh cow's milk for dry skin, absorbs perspiration and keeps skin cool. If excess oil is a problem, water is added to the powder together with a little black tamarind, processed to reduce its excessive acidity, which removes excess oil and closes the pores. Today there are shop-bought equivalents of the same product.

Other treatments include a full complement of natural body peeling powders, scrub lotions, oils and hand creams, breast treatments, shampoos and conditioners, not to mention the Indonesian cosmetics themselves. Ingredients for these run the whole gamut from fruit and vegetables to herbs and spices. One finds no less than nine kinds of ginger, lemons, lime, carrots, spinach, celery, rice, coconuts, oranges, aloe vera, ylang-ylang and roses, as well as copious amounts of betel leaves, tamarind, eggs, honey and sandalwood in such products.

The Most Popular Ingredients

In all, 64 species of plants are used in traditional cosmetics, which can be divided into five groups: face, beauty, hair, body care and medicated cosmetics. Nearly all double as medicines. The various gingers are by far the most frequently used ingredients in face products and medicated cosmetics; turmeric is a favourite for body care and often also appears in medicated cosmetics.

Urang-aring (false daisy; *Eclipta prostrata*) was used by Indian women as early as AD 600. Indonesians most likely adopted the Indian method of pounding its leaves with coconut oil to produce a hair tonic that stimulates growth and prevents greying. It is also excellent for skin complaints, breathing problems and liver disease. *Remujung* (cat's whiskers; *Orthosiphon aristatus*) and *daun sendok* (rat tail; *Plantago major*) are anti-inflammatory astringents that dry, tone and cleanse, and thus are perfect for skin care products that eliminate pimples. Medically, they are used for bladder complaints and for purifying the blood. Rat tail is often recommended for wounds and bites.

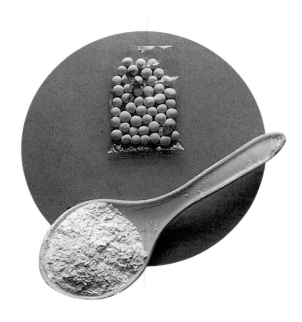

The root of *tapak liman* (*Elephantopus scaber*; prickly-leaved elephant's foot) is a remedy for boils, while chemical components in the leaves are useful for treating chronic diarrhoea and fever. However, it is better known as an aphrodisiac and is used in powders for firming the breasts, which allows it to fall into both medical and beauty treatment categories.

Indonesia's supply of valuable plants is shrinking along with her forests. At least ten important trees and wild plants may soon disappear as a result of logging and the slash-and-burn farming methods. These include plants like sandalwood, *jenitri* (laurel or *Elæocarpus ganitrus*), *sidowayah* (Grandchild's arrival or *Woodfordia fruticosa*), *kayu rapet* (*Parameria lævigata*, a woody climber), *seprantu* (prickly disk or *Sindora sumatrana/javanica*) and *patmosari* (*Rafflesia patma*). All are used in many beauty products both for their active ingredients and their scents.

Sandalwood gives a wonderful, heady scent to cosmetic powders and perfumes; Western aromatherapists recommend it for its tranquil effect, while oil distilled from the bark is used to boost the sex drive of men and women. It is also good for fevers and vomiting. Unfortunately, Indonesia's sandalwood is becoming very scarce, and as the tree must be ten years old before it is felled, this makes future supplies uncertain. The *patmosari* (the gigantic Rafflesia) has a reputation as a powerful female aphrodisiac, but it is often drunk for purifying the uterus after childbirth and getting the abdomen back in shape.

Even cosmetic and perfume ingredients like jasmine and patchouli have medical properties. Both are known to lift depression and help cure frigidity or impotence. The smell of ylang-ylang or *kenanga* (*Canangium odoratum*) is equally

Above:
Rice powder, sold in packets of small, hard balls, is ground to a powder and mixed with water to form a cooling face mask.

Ginggang's Reputation

A few hundred metres from the Paku Alam Palace in Yogyakarta stands one of the most famous jamu shops in Indonesia. Called 'Ginggang', the shop is owned by Ibu Subari, daughter of its well-known founder, Ibu Puspumadyo, who started life as one of the workers in Paku Alam Palace. Every day she made jamu for the Sultan, his wife and close members of the royal family, and Paku Alam V personally nicknamed her 'Ginggang'. After the Sultan's death, she continued to make jamu for the royal family. During her years at the palace, the Prince, now Paku Alam VIII, became very ill and Ginggang nursed him back to health with special jamu.

Following the prince's recovery, Ibu Puspumadyo gained a reputation as a healer, so starting a jamu shop was a natural progression. Around 1925 she bought an old stable near the palace and slowly turned it into a café-style jamu shop. Ginggang's finally opened for business in 1940. Her daughter and son-in-law now run the shop. It opens at 8.30 am for 12 hours each day, and still sells the formulæ Ibu Puspumadyo started in the palace.

Ginggang's is large and airy, with an open front overlooking a tree-lined street. The atmosphere is strangely akin to a French sidewalk café, except the smell of herbs replaces that of strong coffee. Large white boards on the yellowing walls list the jamu on sale together with prices. Ibu Supari makes and sells 31 kinds of dried mixtures or jamu *godog*. "My mother used to sell 36 jamu, but we decided to drop five because they had a laxative effect. They cleaned out the stomach efficiently, but having read some of the recently published books and magazines, I didn't think this was too healthy so we stopped them. For the same reason I always tell customers to steam herbs, not boil them. That way they don't lose their goodness."

She sells the same jamu, in what Ginggang term their instant range, for customers who want a drink on the spot. This is made on the premises by her staff of 20 and includes the usual mixtures plus a few special recipes. In the mid 1980s, Ginggang's received an unsolicited testimonial in a paper presented by Dra Harini Sangat-Roemantyo, Senior Researcher at the National Institute of Botanical Research, which stated: "The fresh Ginggang jamu is very effective for several diseases—coughs, flu, fever, stomach problems and stomach ache."

The clean, tidy kitchen is part of the shop, which means customers can watch all the preparations and see large pans of jamu brewing on the stoves. The staff serve 150 people a day with most of the business being done between 5 pm and 7 pm.

The business runs like clockwork. Wasn't there anything that went wrong occasionally? "Not really," we were told, "but if there are lots of customers we sometimes run short of eggs."

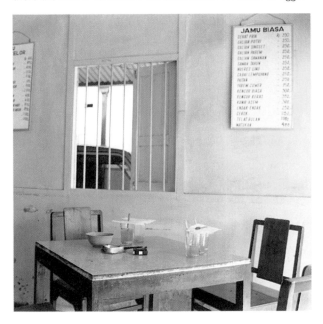

effective sexually because it encourages relaxation and is an excellent tonic for the nervous system. Similarly, Asian belief and Western medical opinion agree that cardamom acts like a magnet on the opposite sex, so perhaps it is not coincidental that it is a popular ingredient in Indonesian cookery.

Shortage of raw materials is not the only factor that has changed traditional cosmetics in recent years. As with international brands, modern marketing has transformed Indonesia's beauty business. Today, many cosmetic powders, creams, eye shadows and lipsticks carry poetic names, such as Thousand Flowers (face powder) or Sunset eyeshadow, to attract both Indonesian customers and intrigue Western ones.

As cosmetic manufacturers combine modern, Western technology with ancient Asian remedies, hopefully they will start to pay more attention to the future of their raw materials. In 1997 alone, the Medicinal Plant Exporters' Association reported that at least 100 species were destroyed by forest fires in Sumatra and Kalimantan. The government recognizes this problem as linked with the general attitude to the environment. In the early 1990s, it approached Professor Koesnadi of Gadjah Mada University to draft Indonesia's new environmental laws, a project he willingly undertook. Its knock-on effect also brings increased Western support for a country that has had, up to now, inadequate environmental policies. To this end, everyone stands to gain.

Jamu and the Burgeoning Spa Industry
Until recently, Europe has been the traditional home of spas, from the original Spa in Belgium to the historical Baden-Baden in Germany and Bath in UK. These began as clinical centres

aimed at curing all types of disease, from arthritis to infertility. Today, the spa concept has shifted emphasis from curing to prevention. We see, worldwide, the rapid growth of spas, ranging in style from 'lean and mean' Californian retreats, to luxurious Southeast Asian resort spas, and quick and easy day spas.

In Indonesia, particularly over the past 10 years or so, the spa boom has been phenomenal. With a focus on spiritual harmony and natural (not pharmaceutical or clinical) treatments, Indonesian spas offer varieties of 'mindful' nourishment—inner and outer beauty and health ritual. It is only natural, therefore, that jamu is also offered. Some spas are run by major jamu producers; others by specialist agencies that have agreed to use specific products; yet others are smaller outfits with just one or two masseurs.

Bali, Indonesia's major tourist destination, offers the visitor a multitude of spa options. Many small hotels, and almost all the larger five-star resorts, have their own spas. Worthy of mention is the spa at Hotel Tugu, a 26-suite type of 'museum boutique hotel' that is overflowing with the owner's collection of antiques. The owner's wife, Dr Wedya Julianti, runs the spa and was responsible for devising the treatment menu of bespoke herbal potions and old-style beauty routines. Specialities include honey face lifting, burnt rice stalks or *merang* to treat grey hair, yoghurt for washing and raw eggs and candlenuts for other therapies. Two other jamu spa companies operating in Bali are Jamu Traditional Spa, KulKulBali, and Jamu-Jamu Traditional Health and Beauty Spas. Both use recipes handed down from generations of Indonesian women, and offer one-off treatments or more substantial three- to five-day retreats. The Begawan Giri

The Ken Dedes Treatment

One of Jakarta's Salon Puri Ayu's most popular indulgences is a Ken Dedes bath. This treatment originated in 13th-century East Java at the court of King Ken Arok, whose wife was renowned for her beauty. It was created exclusively for women and is specially recommended for brides who wish to add extra zing to their sex lives.

The treatment begins with a *kenanga* oil massage. Next comes the aromatic body steam, followed by a bath with *mangir* herbal soap to lighten the skin. This is followed by a leisurely soak in secret, aromatic spices and when this is finished, there is yet another bath in exotic flowers. The final touch is a *ratus* body perfuming using fragrant smoke. This minimizes perspiration, eliminates discharge and give the body a fragrance that smells heavenly for hours.

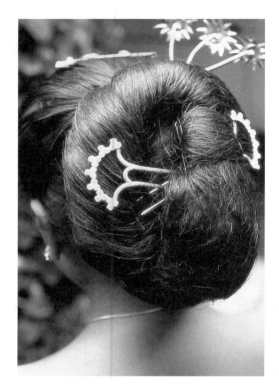

Above:
The complicated and exotic hair styles embellished with gold combs and pins are standard practice for a Javanese bride at her wedding. On that one special event she is supposed to resemble a queen for the day.

Estate spa is unusual because it is set in the open, alongside a cascading holy stream that runs through the grounds. Another day spa of particular note is the Bodyworks Centre in Ubud. Run by well-known healer Ketut Arsana, it specializes in healing massage with Balinese traditional oils, and also offers reflexology, deep tissue massage, acupressure, Swedish techniques and skin exfoliation treatments for removal of toxins.

A popular choice in many spas is the Dewi Sri Spa range of body scrubs, lotions and oils created by Martha Tilaar. Based on traditional ingredients used by princesses in the palaces of Central Java (Dewi Sri is the Indonesian Goddess of Rice), this specialist range is also retailed internationally. Esens, another range of products used extensively in Bali, is concocted by Cary and Kim Collier, spa consultants who have spent years researching the natural health remedies of Indonesia. Their success led the Colliers to introduce their products to the American market in 1999. Called JAMU Inc., Asian Spa Rituals, response has been very positive. "The reverence for nature, the cultivating of the *apotik hidup*, the indigenous knowledge that lives in each Indonesian family, is supported here in the USA," notes Kim Collier. "We focus on both the external (*lulurs*, *borehs*, clay and salts) and the internal (jamu elixirs to complement each jamu ritual)."

The list of spas is endless. But what all of these companies have in common is the ambition to provide a serene atmosphere and stress-busting treatments for weary minds, bodies and souls. One thing is certain: whatever the treatment selected, it will certainly be offered in the spirit of ancient health and beauty practices.

Jamu Darmi: A Small but Important Player

Jamu Darmi is a cottage industry housed in an old residence in a suburb of Central Jakarta. Its range of herbal medicines is no different from many others, but its founder, Ibu Sri Soedarmilah Soeparto, is what makes the business exceptional.

Soedarmilah was reading medicine at Airlangga University, Surabaya, when her studies were halted due to the Japanese invasion. She married and raised a family, but also read widely on health issues. Developing an interest in herbal medicine, she became familiar with the works of Heyne and Kloppenburg-Versteegh. After a while, she developed into something of an expert herbalist. In 1965, at the age of 45, Soedarmilah became a herbal medicine consultant for the huge Sarinah Department Store, in Jakarta, in which jamu products risked being replaced by modern drugs. The promotion was a success and before long Ibu Soeparto was asked to appear on television. Soon, she was presenting her own health programme, with doctors, physicians and pharmacists as guests. She also wrote books and papers on jamu and was frequently invited to speak at international medical conferences. Because of the exposure and increased business, in 1968 Ibu Soeparto was able to set up Jamu Darmi, producing various herbal products exclusively for Sarinah. The company established itself as the industry leader when it pioneered the production of jamu in capsule form, which eliminated the notorious bitter taste. Ibu Soeparto was also among the first to realize that many foreigners wished to return to traditional medicine, and thus strove to open up markets worldwide. Later, Ibu Soeparto started her own plantation about 30 km south of Jakarta near Bogor, as she wanted to control the quality and supply of raw materials that were difficult to find.

In late 1981, Ibu Soeparto was involved in a government scheme to set up a school in which doctors and jamu manufacturers could exchange ideas and information. Lecturers for a two-month course were drawn from the medical profession as well as the body of jamu producers and those in related specialist fields. Topics ranged from hygiene and community health to jamu making and botany, and from traditional massage to laws and rules regulating drug making. In 1983, three groups of students successfully completed their training. Unfortunately, the course was later discontinued.

Not relishing the prospect of repaying huge bank loans, Ibu Soeparto did not want to build a major company. Instead, she channelled her energies into health education programmes and promoted jamu with near missionary zeal. As a former medical student, Ibu Soeparto was aware that herbal medicines must be used with care. She thus recommended it should not be prescribed to treat certain diseases, but otherwise advocated jamu whole-heartedly for over 40 common ailments, including congenital abnormalities, serious shortage of vitamins, cancer and tumours, infections and contagious diseases, metabolic diseases, acute heart and liver complaints, heavy bleeding, neurosis, asthma and schizophrenia.

Her professionalism, single-mindedness and technical knowledge have changed people's perceptions towards jamu. Thanks to her efforts and those of other like-minded pioneers, the jamu industry has now begun to take off internationally.

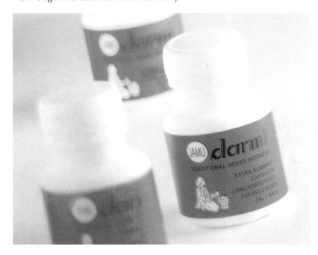

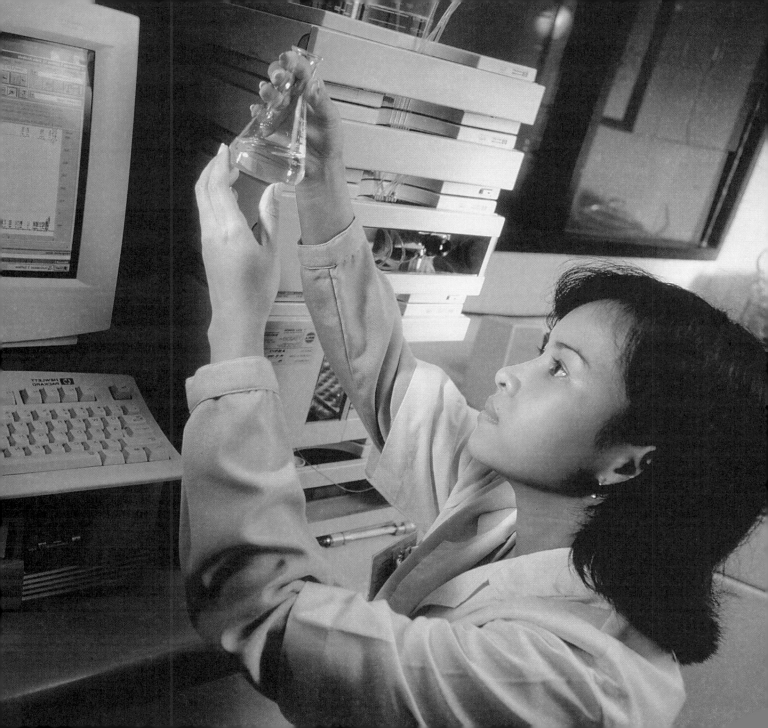

Chapter 7. The Industry

By the 1980s, a few medium sized jamu producers had grown sufficiently to introduce large-scale, modern production methods. Ten years later, Indonesia's jamu industry comprised around 500 companies, including 20 major players.

Left:
The modern factory laboratory of today's health and beauty industry in Indonesia where quality controllers and well trained scientists implement checks that more than equal their western counterparts. Photo courtesy of Martina Berto.

Making and selling jamu was very much a one-man (or, more usually, a one-woman) show until the beginning of the 20th century. A few jamu makers, aware of the increasing demand for jamu and perhaps aware of potential profits, began making and selling in larger quantities. As word spread of their jamu's quality and effectiveness, they were inundated with orders and Indonesia's herbal medicine sprouted a cottage industry.

In the post-war, and indeed post-colonial, years the government backed plans to put jamu on a better footing. There was a need for standardization and for government endorsement if the cottage industry was to shrug off its grassroots tag and move with the times. To this end, five research centres were set up in Indonesia, institutes that set out the criteria for the industry today. By the 1980s, a few medium-sized jamu producers had grown sufficiently to introduce large-scale, modern production methods. In addition, new companies were developed that followed a similar style. Ten years later, Indonesia's jamu industry comprised around 500 companies, including 20 major players.

Looking for a Diabetes Cure

West Sumatran pharmacist Drs Munir studied pharmacy at the prestigious Gadjah Mada University and worked at the Department of Health in Jakarta for many years. Over 15 years ago, he was diagnosed as a diabetic.

After comparing the traditional versus orthodox approach, Drs Munir chose jamu and systematically worked through several traditional medicines. Many either had negative side effects or did not work; he eliminated *daun bangkuwang* (yam bean leaves), seeds of the Java plum, *daun jengkol* (leaves of *Pithecellobium jiringa* tree) and black rice.

Then an old university friend introduced Podosalametee, which was recommended by the Department of Health. He decided to try it and ten days later his blood sugar levels dropped from 210 to a healthy 83. He now takes 20 pills three times a day after meals and adjusts the dosage according to a daily urine test done with glucose sticks. If they turn blue he only takes five to ten pills.

"I was always exhausted before taking this jamu," he says, thrilled. "But now I can even drive myself to Sumatra without any problem."

As a qualified pharmacist what made Drs Munir choose jamu? "With my background I know exactly what goes into Western drugs and what their effects are. That's why I feel much safer with jamu. I'm happy to take Bodrex or Paracetamol for colds, flu or a bit of a temperature but for something long term, I want medicine I can trust, like Podosalametee."

Without a doubt, the top five companies are Jamu Air Mancur, Jamu Jago, Martina Berto, Mustika Ratu and Nyonya Meneer. A combination of dynamic management, modern marketing and the latest technology has made them leaders in the herbal medicine field. They are all forward-thinking, award-winning companies. As it is impossible to include them all, Martina Berto has been chosen to represent the group.

Martina Berto is frequently cited as a model for the jamu industry owing to its outstanding standards of production, retailing, training and management. Like other prominent companies, Martina Berto has been instrumental in redefining jamu in Indonesia by supplying it in a convenient form, not just throughout the country, but beyond its borders. This has made business easier for some of her smaller competitors, but essentially it has served to publicize the values of traditional healing in places where it was formerly regarded with suspicion.

Current Production

Although jamu has been a popular dietary supplement in Indonesia for centuries, especially in Java, times are changing. Young Indonesians are assimilating Western ideas, which include eating convenience foods and taking Western medicines. Many prefer these to drinking the original bitter brews that require aromatic plants to disguise unpleasant smells or tastes. To try to make jamu more palatable, manufacturers are working on both quantity of dose, and taste. The usual dose for manufactured jamu is ten pills, three times a day. While each pill is tiny, people balk at the quantity and given the choice between swallowing ten pills or pellets, a capsule or tablet (one tablet is equal in size to six or seven pills), they go for the easy option. Since these are made from concentrated herbal extracts, a smaller dose achieves the same result.

The jamu industry is also changing as major players have their eye on lucrative international markets. As part of Martina Berto's export strategy the company entered a nine-month assessment programme which led to ISO 9001 certification by the International Accreditation Association of England; it was also awarded NAC-CB and ANSI-RAB in the United States, prestigious awards for any company.

The company manufactures to a Standard System of Quality that is continuously revised and improved. Each department involved in manufacturing has introduced its own operations system and set procedures, which ensure production is fully standardized. For instance, there are strict standards for each raw material, formula, half-finished and finished products, as well as packaging materials. The same applies to raw material cleaning procedures, processing products and storage. Production may be summed up as follows:

Preparation of raw materials:
 – Cleaning with water to wash off any remaining soil;
 – Drying in an oven until they contain less than 10 per cent humidity;
 – Storing in a jamu warehouse: hygiene and air-conditioning are important as they maintain the correct level of humidity. Many raw materials have already reached this stage when they arrive at the factories but some need to go through the preparation outlined above.

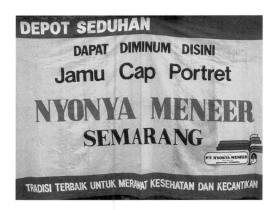

Above:
A banner advertising Nyonya Meneer jam is displayed at small stalls and shops throughout the country. It says that it may be drunk on the premises which is often a wooden bench beside a table where the products are stacked in packets ready to be made up.

Manufacture of product
– Weighing of raw materials according to the formula;
– Mixing;
– Grinding;
– Extracting;
– Finished product: the mixture is made into pills, capsules, tablets or packaged in powder form.

Demand determines the quantity produced and in what form. Adjusting the format is easy because basic formulæ for each product type are the same.

Quality Control of Finished Product

The jamu industry is plagued by accusations concerning its lack of hygiene and efficient quality control techniques. In some cases this criticism may be justified, but all the major firms respect this aspect of production and are fully aware that mistakes could have dire consequences in terms of patient health and their own credibility.

The Quality Control Department at Martina Berto, for instance, has its own operational procedure for inspecting all incoming and outgoing goods according to standards set by the Research and Development Department. The former is responsible for validating production machinery, instruments and equipment, and checking micro-organism levels in the product. Its brief includes monitoring hygiene during production and setting procedures for sanitizing equipment and processing areas.

In such factories, high standards of quality and uniformity are achieved by standard checking systems built into the production flow, which snap into action when random testing is carried out on the finished product to check the microbial count and level of pathogenic micro-organisms. If results exceed the allowed amount, the product is either reprocessed or rejected. Quality controllers carry out an identification check on each delivery of raw materials by eye and under the microscope.

The Research and Development Department has also set standards for every raw material. In technical terms this involves macroscopic, morphologic and microscopic analysis as well as checking ash content or aqueous and alcoholic extract content. Having developed a product, the Research and Development Department is responsible for supervising its manufacture until the production team is satisfied they no longer need this backup. Even so, the Research and Development Department is on hand to iron out any manufacturing problems that may arise in the future. These are very different from the analyses required for chemical drugs, but at present there is no requirement to pinpoint the active ingredients in raw materials. Furthermore, the complexity and large number of active substances in plants mean the majority of properties have not yet been identified.

Maintaining Quality Outside the Factory
Ideally jamu should be stored in clean, dry, cool conditions, away from direct sunlight. Reputable manufacturers always ensure packaging is tightly sealed to protect contents from moisture and humidity. Since they are organic, jamu ingredients are easily contaminated. For instance, if jamu becomes too wet, mould appears. This explains why moisture is carefully controlled during production; were this overlooked, large quantities of

jamu would not reach the customer in good condition. In addition, international standards for hardness and disintegration time (the time it takes for tablets to dissolve in the stomach) are laid down for jamu pills and tablets.

New Directions
As companies look to the future, new products are appearing. For example, the growing demand for health foods has encouraged manufacturers to develop herbal products that may also be classified as food. These include teas for slimming, relaxation, fluid retention and the common cold.

In recent years the upsurge of interest in aromatherapy and spa treatments has led Martina Berto to develop Oil of Java, a range of pure essential oils with exotic Indonesian scents. They are also used in its Dewi Sri Spa range, which combines rice and essential oils to make a variety of tantalizing products.

Jamu Shops
Once it leaves the factories, jamu is available to the retailer through various outlets. Chic department stores carry jamu. Sarinah Department Store, for instance, was instrumental in the creation of Jamu Darmi (see page 157). Nyonya Meneer has its own store in Bali. The larger supermarkets carry a supply while smaller shops may sell jamu along with other products; in certain parts of the country there are stores specializing in jamu.

The Indonesian jamu shop is ubiquitous, but is concentrated in regions with a strong tradition in herbal medicine, the expertise, raw materials and, of course, customers who have been taking jamu since they were born. Large and varied

Profile of an Industry Giant

From an idea in the early 1970s, Dr Martha Tilaar built up one of Indonesia's most important herbal medicine and cosmetics companies, Martina Berto. Today, the Martina Berto Group employs over 6,000 people and has a very healthy turnover.

Dr Tilaar recognized the essence of jamu is its simplicity. Jamu keeps the body in perfect health while the massages, lotions and cosmetics enhance it. This fusion of health and beauty, an age-old philosophy, is the linchpin of Dr Tilaar's vision. Combining natural ingredients with modern research and production techniques, and strict quality control, she launched the product range, Sari Ayu, in 1974, and brought her concept of inner beauty to Indonesian women. It was an unqualified success.

In 1981, Dr Tilaar constructed a factory, which was state of the art for the fledgling industry. Its standards of hygiene held their own with the West's best. Today the Group has three huge factories that operate to the highest technical and scientific standards. As testimony to Dr Tilaar's dedication, Martina Berto has received an impressive number of awards, including the Asia Award for Quality, the American Gold Star Award for Quality and—twice—the International Trophy for Quality. The company's Centre for Non Formal Education in Beauty and Health Care was also recognized when it won the Government National Trophy for the best school of its kind in Indonesia. Because of its prime position in Indonesian business, Dr Tilaar is frequently invited to lecture at management and business meetings throughout the world.

The company is constantly expanding. Current activities include the production of cosmetics, herbal medicines and food supplements, and the operation of four beauty schools and 25 beauty salons in Indonesia. Further salons have been opened in Pakistan, Brunei and the USA. Martina Berto makes over 400 health and beauty products concentrated under four main brands: Sari Ayu herbal cosmetics, Martina Herbal Products, Pesona Indonesian cosmetics and Biokos Total Age Care, a rejuvenating skincare range designed both for Asian and Caucasian women. It also produces Indonesian aromatherapy care and Dewi Sri spa products. The company also runs a foundation course for jamu research, training programmes for *jamu gendong* and organizes lavish enactments of traditional ceremonies, such as royal weddings. Staging these events may be very expensive, but they generate massive press and television coverage, thus ensuring the scheme is cost effective.

These glittering media events also fulfill another equally important purpose: they preserve Indonesia's unique cultural heritage—which is rapidly disappearing—an issue Dr Tilaar feels strongly about. As part of this effort, the company liaises closely with the Ministry of Education and Culture to distribute videos of these impressive events throughout Indonesia's school system. Future plans include dozens of salons worldwide and the formation of its own MBA course for female graduates. Those who complete their studies will have the opportunity to become involved with the international management team of the company. *(Photo courtesy of Martina Berto.)*

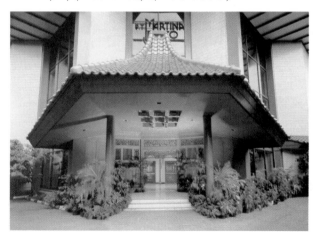

Health Notes

Tests conducted at Widya Mandala University, Surabaya, on jamu supplied by *jamu gendong* in markets around Surabaya, revealed that 80 per cent of the potions were below the Department of Health standards. The researchers concluded that incorrectly stored raw materials and lack of clean water were responsible for this high level of contamination. Whilst most *jamu gendong* would be slighted if you cast doubts on the safety of their products, others, usually through ignorance, do not always apply the same diligence to their ingredients and jamu. It is, therefore, always wisest to visit a well-respected and personally recommended *jamu gendong*.

populations in cities such as Jakarta, Surabaya, Bandung and Yogyakarta result in a high demand for jamu. Universities here have designated centres for jamu research and clinical trials, thereby publicizing the benefits of traditional medicine. Bogor, south of Jakarta, is a special case because its cooler climate is ideal for growing medicinal plants. Ironically, few Sundanese who live in the area know much about making jamu.

Solo, Yogyakarta, Semarang and Surabaya are big jamu centres. People in both Central and East Java have inherited herbal medicine skills, so jamu shops are extremely common in Solo and Yogyakarta. These shops stay open late into the night and usually sell fresh as well as packaged jamu. Would-be jamu buyers are aware that whatever their size, style or location, jamu shops in most cities attempt to come up with a sensible answer to a health problem. In some places, one brand of jamu is sold exclusively. For instance, Cap Jago jamu products are sold at a busy outlet in Solo that resembles a juice bar. The atmosphere is very social and drinks are served into the small hours. Another shop, Akar Sari, is owned by a small factory on the outskirts of Solo. This shop successfully blends modern retailing with the jamu tradition; its open front, displaying all its wares, helps attract customers.

Market Sales

On a grassroots level, jamu sells very well. Some of the smaller outlets—kiosks or market stalls—sell the pre-packed, powdered version of jamu formulæ, while others mix the contents with water and add a few extras like fresh *kampung* eggs or pure wild honey, and as many again sell their own home-made jamu.

A good jamu shop in a city market will carry a huge stock of factory-made pills and powders, which, along with its own jamu, are briskly sold in the course of the day. Many jamu retailers are from Central Java and have been immersed in the jamu culture since birth; others learn from experience acquired on the job. Most know their business thoroughly and hand out good advice.

Markets are the main source of jamu raw materials and the one at Jalan Pintu Besar in Jakarta's Chinatown is by far the largest supplier to the trade. Although Central Java is considered the heart of the industry, this huge market is regarded as a wholesaler to many small jamu producers all over the country. Jakarta's prosaically-named Blok A is typical of the busy, city markets. Inside the building it is hot, stuffy and overcrowded day long. Stalls are numbered but are always referred to by the owner's name, and have different opening and closing hours, though most retailers are open between 10 am and 4 pm. It is hard to gauge exactly which products sell best, but the jamu seller has a comprehensive range of pre-packed cures for all but the most severe or rare illnesses. Nyonya Meneer, Cap Jago, Simona: all the big names are stocked.

Most stores pack maximum products into minimum space. Some vendors can even make up jamu for clients using formulæ which comprise 35 different spices while the range of raw materials necessary may be even wider. A good jamu seller may also supply local *jamu gendong* with their basic materials, which are then taken home and used in their own preparations. As with *jamu gendong*, service in the markets is friendly and personal and the sellers are well-informed—something that people prefer when discussing their health.

The Sum of the Parts

American scientists recently conducted some interesting herbal experiments whereby they extracted five compounds from a number of herbs normally used in a specific jamu and fed them separately to animals.

When the progress of this group was compared with that of other animals which had been fed a mixture containing all the compounds, results clearly showed that when taken individually none of the compounds had any effect. However, the health of animals eating the combination of five compounds improved dramatically over the testing period.

Similar tests were carried out with a control group of people, who took a placebo, and a second group, who were prescribed jamu. Reaction proved positive in the group taking jamu. Whilst useful, such tests are unfortunately not sufficient to give this jamu its scientific credentials.

A High Profile Business Woman

Martha Tilaar was born in Kebumen, Central Java, to a family of wealthy landowners whose business interests ranged from beef and butcheries to dairy farming and dairies. Such privileged circumstances ought to have been the basis of a happy childhood but Martha Tilaar's early years were not story-book perfect.

"I was always considered the black swan of the family. My brother and sister were fair while I was dark. My features were totally different too—I didn't look like any of them." Martha responded by ignoring anything to do with her looks. Instead, she became known for her tomboy attitude and rebellious behaviour.

After she finished school, Martha went to a teacher training college in Jakarta, which was over 550 km (300 miles) from home. But at the start of her first teaching job, her mother intervened, intent on improving her daughter's appearance. She took the girl to the home of a friend who was a beautician, for a consultation that was to change not only the young woman's attitudes but also her future. "Until that moment, I didn't care about beauty at all," she said. "But when I was shown what to do and saw the difference a few professional touches made, I was convinced." Thus, from shunning beauty treatments and cosmetics, Martha became an aficionado.

Today, she is an extremely attractive woman in her early sixties. Those who meet her for the first time invariably remark on her flawless skin, impeccable grooming, personal style and magnetism. Her transition from teacher to tycoon began in 1964, when Martha Tilaar married a fellow teacher. The comfortable life she had previously taken for granted evaporated as the reality of life married to an academic set in. Although Alex Tilaar soon accepted a prestigious five-year scholarship in education and philosophy in the States, the financial situation changed little. Martha, however, began working as a child minder to married students with families. Once she had managed to save sufficient money, she enrolled in a course at Bloomington's Academy of Beauty Culture. To help cover costs, she worked as an Avon lady in her spare time, selling cosmetics door-to-door. It was a tough learning curve, but when she graduated in 1968, Martha Tilaar had mastered the skills necessary to start her own beauty business. Jakarta in the 1970s, she felt, was ready for a Western-style beauty salon.

The salon she created was far removed from Jakarta's norm. Air conditioning, hot and cold running water, and an American approach ensured Jakarta's elite boosted Martha Tilaar's burgeoning business. Clearly, she had found her métier. The temptation to expand was irresistible. Beauty is a volatile market and the fledgling entrepreneur knew if she wanted her business to grow, she would soon have to review her strategy. For this purpose, she took a trip to Europe where she met Dutch cosmetologist, Dr Van Der Hoog, who convinced her that the 'back-to-nature' movement was the cosmetic trend of the future. He further pointed out that Indonesia had the finest store of natural ingredients in the world. Martha realized that the resources, and the markets, were indeed in her own country.

At the same time, after years of trying for a baby, and having resorted to the use of jamu over a few years, Martha discovered she was pregnant at last. Where modern gynæcology had been unable to help, homespun jamu had proven successful. A second child soon followed. As with many other modern Indonesian women, the new mother began to re-evaluate the medicine of her ancestors, but was initially thwarted by the stigma attached to it. The prevailing attitude was summed up by a wealthy society lady: "My driver goes to the shop every morning and buys me a glass of fresh jamu but I always drink it in the car where no one can see me."

Martha Tilaar's problem was how to improve commercial jamu's image. Steeped in mystery, celebrated for its culture, mystic traditions, the elegance and legendary beauty of royal women, the life in Javanese royal courts is still regarded with awe and wonder by Indonesians and foreigners alike. Martha Tilaar thus realized that if jamu had an association with the ancient palaces of Central Java, it would gain prestige.

However, the formulæ responsible for royal beauty were closely guarded and kept strictly within palace walls. Martha Tilaar sought an audience with the Queen of Mangkoenegoro Palace in Solo to plead her case and became the first person outside royal circles to be entrusted with the much coveted secret formulæ. After a year of intense experimentation, she was ready to launch the new range, named Sari Ayu, or Essence of Beauty. Despite her efforts, the product was not an instant success; preconceptions concerning home-made and budget priced products were among factors that deterred sales.

Further research took Martha Tilaar to the palace of Sri Sultan Hamengku Buwono IX in Yogyakarta, where she spent hours poring over ancient Javanese manuscripts. She learned that for generations Javanese court ladies had followed a total health and beauty regime based on the concept of Rupasampat Wahya Bhiantara, inner and outer beauty. "In Indonesia beauty is brought out from the inside. A woman does not have to be born beautiful to be beautiful, but she must know how to bring out her beauty." This was the key to repositioning Sari Ayu.

This change proved to be successful and in 1981 Martha Tilaar opened her first factory, today considered a model for the blossoming industry. Her vision was to re-create tradition but this time by combining natural ingredients with modern research, production techniques and strict quality control. Based on these principles, Sari Ayu took Total Beauty straight out of history and presented it to the women of Indonesia. Brilliant, romantic, magical—no wonder they clamoured for it. Demand overtook supply overnight and her order books overflowed.

Despite the amazing success of her business, Martha Tilaar still pushes herself to the limit. Her working day starts when she picks up the phone at 7 am and does not usually finish until late into the evening. When she travels, she puts herself through a punishing schedule for the cause of beauty and for Martina Berto, the name of the company which now produces the Sari Ayu line. Her involvement is total, her enthusiasm infectious and her working hours unlimited. But Ibu Martha simply shrugs and says: "I am in love with this business."

If you listen to gossip you will find that the name Martha Tilaar is either loved or feared, that there are no half measures. In some circles she is known as 'the godmother'. In business she is said to be dynamic, driven and uncompromising. Indeed, she says of herself, "I am very, very tough", and has proven this quality repeatedly. People close to Ibu Martha speak of her leadership qualities, personal charisma, warmth and sense of fun. In private, she is said to be very emotional and kind-hearted, although this softer side is carefully kept under wraps.

It is typical that on weekends she often goes off on her own to collect handicrafts and batiks from the villages. The generous gesture is dismissed with "they're so poor someone has to help them". Staff are used to receiving an assortment of goods to be promoted and sold. Such adventures can have unusual results: one day a whole factory corridor was festooned with beautifully made paper lanterns. They were apparently the work of an 80-year-old woman who was almost destitute. To help, Ibu Martha bought her entire stock, then faced the problem of what to do with it.
(Photo courtesy of Martina Berto.)

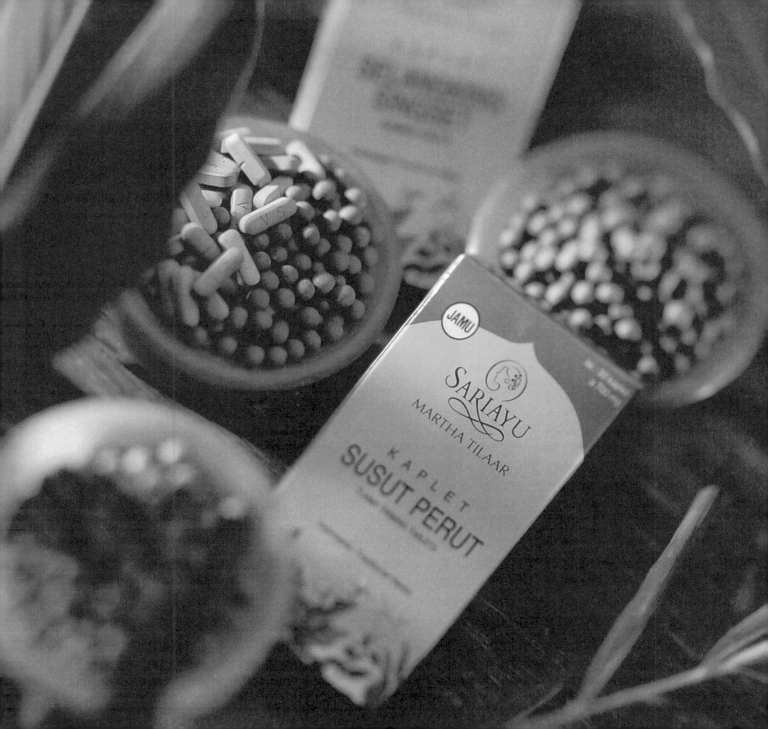

Chapter 8. The Way Ahead

As the media and the internet contribute towards improving awareness of health and fitness, patients are becoming more knowledgeable. Holistic medicine is on the upsurge.

Left:
Factory-made jamu products available over the counter in the form of pills and capsules or powders.
(Photo courtesy of Martina Berto.)

Indonesian traditional medicine has survived centuries of change and, despite the advent of modern medicine, latest estimates from the Department of Health reveal that 49 per cent of the population continue to drink herbal remedies. Indonesian manufacturers are now looking at ways of expanding their markets and introducing different types of herbal based products. Examples of these are packaged drinks sold under the health banner. They still use jamu as their unique selling point and have turned its magic appeal to advantage.

In September 1995, an Asian Wall Street Journal editorial related that Indonesians still equate jamu with health. The newspaper documented the extraordinary success of Refreshing Solution, a packaged drink that looks and tastes like water. Refreshing Solution claims to both cure and prevent "mouth ulcers, sore throats, constipation and what Indonesians call *panas dalam* (internal body heat)".

Refreshing Solution was originally launched in the mid-1980s but had little impact until 1994, when its makers launched an intensive two-year television campaign. According to Indonesian business magazine, SMA, when the campaign finished, the profits from sales of Refreshing Solution were running into US$45 million dollars.

Why has such a product acquired so many avid fans? The *Asian Wall Street Journal* points out that Refreshing Solution's "lack of flavour is not to everyone's taste", but goes on to say: "The manufacturer made a shrewd move to appeal to many different groups of Indonesians by putting the word jamu on the label. The SMA article picked up on this point by congratulating Mr Budi Yuwono of Sinde Budi Sentosa who make the drink for being 'brave' to label his drink a traditional medicine. This is exactly what other makers avoid, preferring their products to be known as medicine." The gamble paid off handsomely, such that Refreshing Solution is now available in strawberry, apple, melon and other flavours.

Jamu has also been given a new twist by another product called Coffee Racik. Add ground cardamom, cumin, Javanese brown sugar, *kencur*, cinnamon and ginger root juice to pure ground coffee and you have the drink that keeps you healthy without the usual bitter jamu taste. Racik actually means 'blending the right ingredients'; the product is known as the answer to colds, tiredness, rheumatics, sore throats and body odour. All this, and delicious coffee too, for a reasonable price.

Such new ideas are not exclusive to the beverage industry. Producers of jamu and cosmetics have been introducing herbal remedies in the form of curing teas in sachets, capsules and tablets. Cosmetic ranges have been developed for problem teenage skins, anti-ageing, anti-wrinkling and with a built-in Sun Protection Factor (SPF). Beauty salons have introduced aromatherapy massage using their own local, aromatherapy oils with tempting ingredients, including ginger, nutmeg, peppermint, lemon, cloves, white cumin, cinnamon, cardamom and fennel, while perfumes are derived from sandalwood, vetiver, roses and ylang-ylang flowers.

Packaging, too, is being given a new look. While advertising literature once appeared only in Bahasa Indonesia, it is now being printed in English as well. Jamu is being prepared for foreign markets and companies are thinking export. Undismayed by the maze of legalities and hurdles like America's Food and Drug Administration control, at least nine companies are exploring overseas markets and are not confining their interests to Asia alone. Two producers have already gone public to finance their export plans.

The directors of Traditional Medicine at the Department of Health have visited Europe and America to study import restrictions and approach regulatory boards. Many countries are suspicious of products that have not been 'scientifically proven'; it matters not that a remedy has been going strong for thousands of years. However, some jamu companies have had limited success in foreign markets.

In the case of the recent aromatherapy boom in the West, it is the public that seems to be leading the trend. Books on aromatheraphy are fast sellers, and numerous training courses have sprung up to teach people about the benefits of this ancient art. However, it is still an unknown quantity in a number of ways. Many essential oils used in aromatherapy have been tested only recently, and the hazards of misapplication or misuse are not readily advertised. Many people are not aware that some oils are dangerous if incorrectly mixed or wrongly applied, and seem to think if something is applied to the skin, it cannot do any harm. It is not common knowledge that one of the body's most efficient transport systems moves oils from the skin's surface into the blood stream.

But where health is concerned, logic doesn't always enter into the argument. Take cinnamon, for example. For years, sports massage therapists considered it essential to their work. Yet the oil derived from cinnamon has been banned in some Western countries owing to its toxicity level. One highly qualified British beautician, aromatherapist and sports massage expert was furious over the decision.

"Problems only arise because we don't understand how to use cinnamon and other potentially toxic herbs correctly in the West," she says. "This kind of thing doesn't arise in Asia where reputable healers know exactly when and how much to use. Why not teach therapists how to use the oil instead of rejecting it?" However, such decisions are having little affect on the overall trend as belief in natural medicines is growing.

The West Looks East
Now that some people in the West are beginning to have reservations about orthodox medicine, medical practitioners are considering the implications of treating the whole person more seriously rather than curing parts of the body in isolation. Doctors are increasingly recommending methods used by our grandparents. Professional bodies are recognizing treatments that used to be labelled alternative (acupuncture, osteopathy and reflexology, for example), while in the United States, a

A Profitable Operation

At 54 years of age, Ibu Mulyono has 30 years of jamu experience to her credit. She describes herself as "an old-fashioned woman" and this is reflected in her jamu making. She insists grinding and crushing are done by hand "to ensure the drinks taste fresh". Ibu Mul used to grow most of the ingredients in her own garden until lack of space made it more practical to buy the items from the market instead. Her shopping list usually comprises kencur, jungrabat (Baeckea frutescens), lemons, turmeric, fenugreek, ginger, tamarind, sintok bark (Cinnamomum sintoc), pulosari (Alyxia stellata) and lastly, a solid block of gula Jawa, Javanese brown sugar.

Jamu preparation starts at 7 pm when the men come home from work. They wash the raw materials and do a first crushing in the lumpang, a large, square grinder, using an outsize pestle about one and a half metres (five feet) long. Within two hours, six pastes are roughly ground ready for the second grinding next morning. Their basic preparations complete, the family collapse into bed for a well-earned five and a half hours' sleep.

They rise at 2.30 am to finish making the jamu. The whole place, including the traditional floor of hard packed earth, is kept scrupulously clean. Two fires glow in the background, casting shadows that flicker round the dimly lit room. Sixty-year-old Bapak Mulyono is usually the first to get going in the mornings. He starts by grinding a mix of raw rice and cloves. He kneels on the floor, building up a steady rhythm with the gandik or pestle, as it moves smoothly back and forth over the flat, rectangular grinding stone. At this point Ibu Mul appears to lend a hand. Before starting work, she carefully places a cloth on her lap to protect her clothes and binds her waist with a piece of strong cloth (called a stagen) to prevent straining the muscles of the back.

Five pairs of practised hands go about their business quietly and efficiently. The whole kitchen has a look of organized chaos. Nothing is hurried, the familiar routine flows smoothly. At intervals someone stops what they are doing to check pans of water on the stove and ensure the flame is not too high. Boiling is essential to eliminate impurities. Ibu Mul is also very particular about cooling mixtures when they come off the fire. The hot liquid is transferred from huge steaming metal pots into plastic basins; if it went directly into the special, thick glass bottles, it would break them. Once full, they are sealed with rolled banana leaves. Cold, boiled water is added to the mixture during its second grinding to make the paste finer and keep the ingredients moist whilst they're being worked. Each paste needs at least 15 minutes continuous grinding and like any experienced cook, Ibu Mul knows when it's finished from the texture and feel.

A typical day's stock is five bottles of Beras Kencur; three bottles of bitter mixtures—considered the most effective; two or three bottles of sugar syrup for sweetness; one bottle of ground raw rice and sugar, one bottle of wejah and plastic bags filled with extra, ground kencur to satisfy individual tastes.

"I like to be in place by 7.15 am," she asserts, "because I don't want to disappoint my regulars." Between 7 am and 11 am, there is a continuous stream of people who stop and buy on their way between the street and market. Her recipes taste delicious and the exchange becomes a social occasion when the women catch up on gossip.

Ibu Mul is illiterate, so she relies on memory for her jamu recipes, but with eyes twinkling, she says: "I know the bank notes and can count which is all that's necessary!"

government sub-committee is considering setting up a properly-funded centre for conducting complementary and alternative medicine research.

As the media and the internet contribute towards improving awareness of health and fitness, patients are becoming more knowledgeable. Preventive and holistic medicine is on the rise; the practice of blindly adhering to orthodox drugs has now lost popularity. Medical herbalists are coming back into fashion as people are increasingly disillusioned with orthodox medicine, for though there is much to be said in favour of modern drugs, they can bring unwelcome side effects and patients are looking elsewhere.

A statement made by the British Medical Council some years ago admitted that a high percentage of diagnoses were inaccurate, but there was nothing to worry about as antibiotics were usually prescribed and they cured 70 per cent of all known illnesses. A decade later, the same elite body is telling doctors to stop over-prescribing antibiotics because excessive use renders the drugs less effective. Given this less than encouraging news, is it any wonder faith in back-to-nature treatments is growing apace?

Scientific proof, however, is a big issue. In Indonesia, debate rages on between the jamu industry and the medical profession. Manufacturers argue the cost of testing is prohibitive, when ranges comprise upwards of 200 items. They also maintain that since people have used certain herbs for generations without harm, the cures cannot be toxic. However, many doctors are not prepared to accept such unsubstantiated evidence without scientific proof. As far back as 1993, a report in *Business Indonesia* stated: "It is clear that clinical testing is precisely what is required for jamu to enter the export market. Even if clinical tests prove their efficacy, jamu needs more than reliable test results to be sold to the Western world. It is currently perceived as a strange elixir with a witches-brew kind of aura about it."

Medical and public concern are justified, but should the lack of formal medical research worry prospective users? Perhaps not; consider this statement made by Vincent Marks, Professor of Clinical Biochemistry at Surrey University and spokesman for Healthwatch: "This lack of research is true of all alternative or complementary medicines, but it's also true of 80 per cent of orthodox medicines. Medical intervention has little effect on most illnesses in the long run—the vast majority of them get better of their own accord."

It is a confusing situation, but increasingly, consumers are being offered more choices. Between 1989 and 1995, British sales of herbal medicine rose by 70 per cent, while sales of herbal medicine (excluding homeopathic treatments) in European Union countries jumped by 30 per cent during the same period.

Ironically, as the West looks to the East to solve its health problems, the reverse occurs in Asia; Indonesians often adopt a starry-eyed attitude towards Western medical care. It has brought great improvement in countless areas, such as the dramatic drop in Indonesia's infant mortality rate; however, in other situations, the tried and tested natural answer is often perfectly adequate—and often cheaper.

In *Megatrend 2000*, John Naisbitt and Patricia Abuderne put forward the hypothesis that a reawakening of traditional culture is inevitable in the 21st century. Many Javanese share this view, as prophesized by Sabdopalon 500 years ago when the

Majapahit kingdom fell. Indonesian psychic and international lawyer, Permadi Satrio Wiwoho sees man at a period of transition. He believes there will be a major change globally because people are growing tired of technology, modern drugs and their side effects. He predicts modern medicine and what is now called traditional medicine will exchange roles. Permadi also points out that having failed to find a cure for AIDS and cancer, Western scientists now believe the answer could lie with two natural herbs currently undergoing tests. One day in the not too distant future, he sees medicine again being accompanied by mantras and prayer.

It is a fact that even without the benefit of expensive modern products, Indonesian women are amazingly well preserved, even after producing large families. Indonesians, including some doctors as well as many foreigners living in Indonesia, swear by jamu. Statistics prove that exports of medicinal plants and traditional medicine have increased substantially. The government is now beginning to take this industry seriously and scientific testing is slowly tipping the scales in favour of jamu and traditional medicine.

Will people living in the West resist this Eastern promise of health and beauty? Westerners who have lived in Indonesia are perhaps atypical. They have seen, experienced and, in most cases, been thoroughly impressed by the curative powers of jamu. They have learned that traditional treatments can work where their own clinically proven drugs have failed. The prognosis for jamu is good, but to successfully put these products on the international map requires a fair amount of education, enthusiasm, tenacity and a substantial marketing budget.

Recently, the creation of websites and e-mail addresses for ordering jamu over the World Wide Web have elicited interest (see page 184). It is certainly facilitating the dissemination of knowledge about jamu and will hopefully make jamu more accessible to new users in this new millennium. Similarly, it is hoped that this book will go some way towards clarification and changing misconceptions.

The final words on this subject rightly belong to the famous herbalist, J T Lembong, who stated: "A medical system persisting for many centuries and bringing relief to so many millions cannot be entirely false. Assuming medical professionals in East and West can set aside their jealousies and work as a team, patients of the future could benefit from the best health service the world has ever known." Hopefully, that day is not far away.

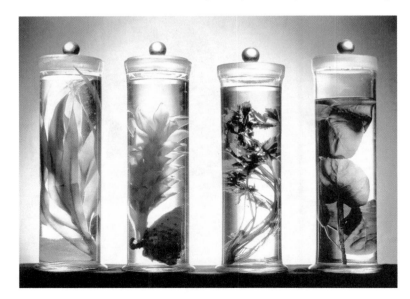

Left:
Storage is one of the most important elements in today's high-tech jamu factories.(Photo courtesy of Martina Berto.)

JAMU

BLUE SINAMON ®

contents : 300 pills @ 150 mg.

To stimulate hair growth

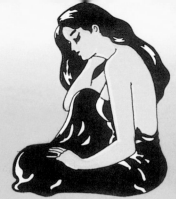

JAMU PILL

Wanita Super

ISI 72 PIL

OBAT
KHUSUS
WANITA

MANJAKANI ®

EURYCOMAE RADIX

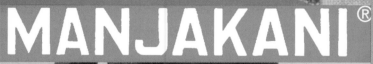

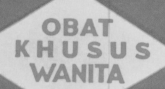

PASAK BUMI

KAPSUL

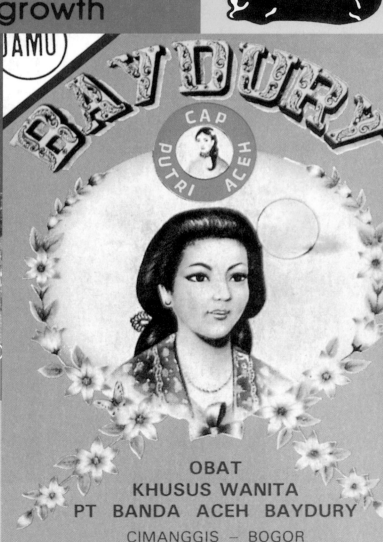

JAMU

BAYDURY

CAP
PUTRI
ACEH

OBAT
KHUSUS WANITA
PT BANDA ACEH BAYDURY

CIMANGGIS – BOGOR

Appendix.

This chapter outlines a number of jamu recipes that have—for the most part—been given to the author by the ordinary Indonesian housewife. Special thanks go to Ibu Atun, Ibu Sujatno, Mbak Sumirah, Mbak Supriyani, Mbak Sriharti and Mbak Sumarsih. Most ingredients are culled from nature's store cupboard, and in cases where fresh Indonesian ingredients are unobtainable or formulæ are complicated, you are advised to buy ready-made products. A tumbler, glass or mug denotes approximately a 50 ml (2 oz) measurement.

Measurements in Indonesia are a mystery. Most jamu makers rely on a mixture of instinct, experience and 'feeling' to gauge just how much of a particular ingredient is required.

To give a first-hand example, when Ibu Sujatno, a traditional masseuse, jamu maker and housewife gave me a recipe for rheumatism massage oil, she simply listed the ingredients: ginger, greater galangal, cloves, lemon grass and coconut oil. She did not specify the quantities. I asked an Indonesian friend, Supriyani, to chase after her and check. When she returned, the list was untouched. I was flummoxed, but Supriyani remained unfazed as she went to the market to buy the five required items and two grated coconuts for making the basic oil. Supriyani set aside $1^{1}/_{2}$ kg of coconut, and deftly divided up the other ingredients. The result was excellent. When asked why she had chosen these amounts, her answer was "I just know".

Left:
Despite huge inroads in the industry, packaging remains traditional on many jamu products.

SIMPLE REMEDIES TO TRY AT HOME

Health

Insomnia

Ingredients: 1 nutmeg mace; 1 mug boiling water

Method: Remove skin from mace of nutmeg. Place skinless mace in a paper or plastic bag and crush with a hammer. Put in a mug and pour boiling water over the top. Allow to stand for at least 30 minutes. Drink before going to bed. If the problem persists after 3/4 days consult a doctor.

To Cool/Treat Spots and Pimples

Ingredients: Jasmine leaves

Method: Wash and pound the jasmine leaves into a paste. Apply to affected areas and leave for 15 minutes. Wash off in warm water followed by rinsing in iced water. Repeat as necessary.

To Avoid Catching Cold

Ingredients: 1 can Sprite lemonade; pinch of salt

Method: Add pinch of salt to a full glass of Sprite and drink before going to bed. Repeat the following night if necessary.

Sore Throat Remedies
Remedy (a)

Ingredients: 50–100 g fresh ginger; 1 1/2 tumblers of water

Method: Peel and slice the ginger into fine strips. Boil in water for 5 minutes. Either strain or pour off the liquid and drink while hot morning and evening till recovered.

Remedy (b)

Ingredients: Juice of lemon or thin-skinned lime (*Jeruk nipis*); 1 dessert spoon light soy sauce

Method: Squeeze the lemon and mix the juice with light soy sauce and drink. Repeat daily.

Cough Remedy

Ingredients: 1 medium sized onion; 1 spoon pure honey and 1/3 local lime (*Jeruk nipis*)

Method: Grate the onion, squeeze the lime and mix the ingredients together. The lime juice and pulp is for binding the other ingredients. If you wish to increase the quantities, triple (never double) the first two items and add to a single lime.

To Treat Wounds

Ingredients: Banana

Method: Mash the banana to a pulp and spread over the wound. Repeat as necessary.

To Reduce Swelling

Ingredients: Old tamarind; salt; small amount of water

Method: Mix the three ingredients to a paste. Massage the affected area daily till the swelling subsides. Can be used for any swelling especially swollen feet.

To Soothe Swollen Gums

Ingredients: Gambier (*Uncaria gambeiri*), extract from tree bark; water

Method: Put gambier in a glass, fill with water and allow to stand for at least 30 minutes. Use as a mouthwash till swelling subsides.

Beras Kencur

General tonic for tiredness; invigorates, improves blood circulation and appetite.

Ingredients: 50 g fresh *kencur*; 50 g raw rice; pinch of salt; knob of tamarind (preferably old Javanese tamarind); brown sugar to taste (preferably Javanese red sugar); 1 cup of water

Method: Allow the raw rice to stand in water for 3 hours. Simmer the sugar in water till fully dissolved. Mix the tamarind with a little warm water and sieve. Peel and cut the *kencur* before grinding with a pestle and mortar till soft together with the softened raw rice.

Mix together all the ingredients; *kencur* ground with raw rice, tamarind, sugar, salt and sieve. The jamu can be drunk warm, but tastes good served chilled with a lump of ice.

Suitable for adults and children over the age of 12 years. Drink a small glass daily or 1 full glass each week.

Kunir Asem

General tonic; with additions, is suitable for treating white vaginal discharge or obesity.

Ingredients: 5 pieces of turmeric (preferably use the grandmother root, i.e. main root. If the roots are small, grate instead of slice); pinch of salt; 2 pieces of tamarind (size of a knob of butter without the seed); palm sugar to taste; 1 1/2 glasses of water

Method for basic recipe: Peel or grate the turmeric depending on its size. Mix with the remaining ingredients, add water and heat in a saucepan till the mixture is just on the boil, remove from heat immediately and leave to cool. Chill in the fridge before drinking. This recipe makes 2 glasses of tonic.

White Vaginal Discharge, Obesity

Ingredients: 5 betel nut leaves

Method: Boil the leaves in water and add liquid to the Kunir Asem basic recipe. Drink the mixture for 3 to 5 days.

For A Sick Stomach

Ingredients: Grandmother root of turmeric; pinch of salt

Method: Peel and grate the grandmother root of turmeric and squeeze out the juice in a piece of clean muslin cloth. Add $1/2$ glass of warm water and drink.

For Stomach Upset/ Bloated Stomach

Ingredients: 2 dessert spoons of red rice (Indonesian *beras merah*); 1 glass of boiling water

Method: Roast (NB: not fry) 2 dessert spoons of rice and put into a glass of boiling water. Leave to stand till the water turns a deep shade of red. Drink once or twice daily till symptoms disappear.

Vitamin B1 is the magic ingredient that helps the curing process.

Rheumatic Massage Oil

Ingredients: 1 $1/2$ kg grated coconut; 175 g *lengkuas*; 175 g fresh ginger; 2 g cloves; 1 tablespoon white pepper; 50 g lemon grass

Method: Mix $1/4$ litre of water into the grated coconut, then sieve the coconut juice into a saucepan. Grind both the *lengkuas* and ginger into a paste in a pestle, about 350 g. Then grind cloves to powder, followed by lemon grass. Add the ground cloves and lemon grass mixture to the *lengkuas* and ginger paste, and stir it, with 1 tablespoon white pepper, into the saucepan.

Boil the mixture on high to medium flame for $2^{1}/4$ hours till the water evaporates and the oil begins to form, stirring frequently to prevent burning. Then, transfer to muslin or fine cotton cloth, and sieve. Leave to drain, and when cool, squeeze hard to extract the liquid. Allow to drain in a sieve overnight to extract any remaining oil. Pour into a glass screw-top bottle for storage.

Beauty
Skin Care
Mask for Soft Skin

Ingredients: Banana

Method: Purée banana in blender, or mash with a fork. Apply to skin especially face, ideally before a bath or shower. Leave for 15 minutes and rinse with warm water. Repeat every 2 to 3 days to keep skin soft.

Mask for Soft, Smooth Skin
Remedy (a)

Ingredients: Tomato

Method: Hand grind or use a blender to make tomato purée. Apply to skin and wash off after 15 minutes. Repeat as necessary.

Remedy (b)

Ingredients: Potato

Method: To clean and soften skin, cut the potato and rub into skin.

Skin Cleanser

Ingredients: Cucumber

Method: To clean skin, wash and slice cucumber. Rub all over skin of face and neck.

Treatment for Blackheads and Spots

Ingredients: Indonesian Rough Green Tea

Method: Make a mug of tea as usual and leave overnight. Wash skin and face with tea water the following morning. Repeat daily.

Healthy Skin

Ingredients: Rice water

Method: Wash skin with rice water i.e. water used to wash raw rice before it is cooked. Prepare by pouring water from the first washing into a glass and allow to stand till fine white powder settles at the bottom of the glass and water becomes clear. Pour off water, leaving nearly a centimetre in the bottom of the tumbler. Cleanse face, stir rice in water and use to rinse face. The vitamins it contains promote healthy skin; it also softens and is very refreshing.

Soft Hands

Ingredients: *Pisang mas* (golden bananas)

Method: Rub hands regularly with the inside of the golden banana skin. This will keep them soft, supple and looking youthful.

Hair tonic

Ingredients: Handful of cananga flowers; 1 glass of coconut oil; handful of jasmine leaves (optional); handful of cup leaves (*Plantago major*—optional)

Method: Boil cananga flowers/cup leaves with the coconut oil and leave to cool. Wash and dry hair. Apply tonic. Use sparingly depending on hair type as too much makes hair oily. Leave on the hair. Hair does not need to be washed again.

REPUTABLE JAMU PRODUCERS IN INDONESIA

PT Berial Sumber Medica
Jalan Mayjend Sungkono 355
Surabaya
East Java
Indonesia
Tel: (62-31) 5662156

PT Dami Sariwana
Jalan Industri Raya Timur II/A-26
Semarang 50111
Central Java
Indonesia
Tel: (62-24) 6580946
Fax: (62-24) 6593688
www.damisariwana-herb.com/main.htm
email: damiherb@damisariwana-herb.com

PT Deltomed Laboratories
Jalan Jenderal Sudirman 158
Wonogiri 51601
Central Java
Indonesia
Tel: (62-273) 22566
Fax: (62-273) 21118

PT Indo-Farma
Jalan Indo Farma No 1
Gandasari
Cibitung
Bekasi 17520
West Java
Indonesia
Tel: (62-21) 8800025, 8800727
Fax: (62-21) 8800029, 8800030

PT Jamu Air Mancur
Ruko Plaza Blok HD 4–6
Jalan Raya Solo Baru 1
Solo Baru
Central Java
Indonesia
Tel: (62-271) 20980, 20981
www.airmancur.co.id

Jaya Raya Solo Sragen KM 7 Palur

P.O. Box 253
Solo 57102
Central Java
Indonesia
Tel: (62-271) 25197, 25024, 26183
Fax: (62-271) 25198

PT Jamu Borobudur
Jalan Sumber MAS I/B-14
Semarang 50178
Central Java
Indonesia
Tel (62-24) 518427
Fax (62-24) 552212
www.jamu-borobudur.com
e-mail: info@jamu-borobudur.com

PT Jamu Darmi
Menteng Dalam RT008/01
No. 30 Pancoran Tebet
Jakarta 12870
Indonesia
Tel: (62-21) 8298521

PT Jamu Iboe Jaya
Jalan Kutai 22
Surabaya 60241
East Java
Indonesia
Tel: (62-31) 5682714, 5680330, 5680645
Fax: (62-31) 567921
www.jamuiboe.com
e-mail: info@jamuiboe.com

PT Jamu Indonesia Simona
Jalan Kompol Maksum 237
Semarang 50242
Central Java
Indonesia
Tel: (62-24) 314878
Fax: (62-24)412835

PT Jamu Jago
Jalan Kimangun Sarkoro 106
Semarang 50136
Central Java
Indonesia
Tel: (62-24) 543800

Fax: (62-24) 547938
www.inc.com/users/jamujago.html
e-mail: jamujago@vision.net.id

PT Jamu Sido Muncul
Jalan Industri 2A No 19
Kaligawe KM4 LIK
Tanah Makmur
Semarang
Central Java
Indonesia
Tel: (62-24) 580559
Fax: (62-24) 580332
email: marketing@sidomuncul.com
www.sidomuncul.com

Jakarta office
Tel: (62-21) 7653535
Fax: (62-21) 7656522

PT Kimia Farma
Jalan Budi Utomo No 1
Jakarta Pusat 10710
Indonesia
Tel: (62-21) 3857243, 3849251
Fax: (62-21) 3441418

Jalan Ir H Juanda No 1
Bandung
Jawa Barat
Indonesia
Tel: (62-22) 4205421

PT Konimex
Desa Sanggrahan
Kecamatan Grogol Sukoharjo
PO Box 233
Surakarta
Indonesia
Tel: (62-271) 36965, 46966, 46246
Fax: (62-271) 46247

Jalan Kenangan 3
Badran
Solo 51702
Indonesia

PT Leo Agung Raya
Kepada Gading Blvd
Blok RA II/21
Jakarta 14240
Indonesia
Tel: (62-21) 4525145

Factory: Jalan Pemuda 23-B
Semarang
Indonesia
Tel: (62-24) 515839, 512283, 661692
Fax: (62-24) 512264

PT Marguna Jarulata
Jalan Hang Tuah 8
Tegal
Indonesia
Tel: (0283) 91707
Fax: (0283) 91768

PT Martina Berto
Jalan Pulokambing II No 1
Kawasan Industri, Pulogadung 13930
Indonesia
Tel: (62-21) 4603717/4603718/4603719
Fax: (62-21) 4606245
www.martha-tilaar.com

PT Maryong Mondo – Jamu Nyonya Marie
Jalan Industri VII 323–325 LIK
Semarang 50111
Indonesia
Tel: (62-24) 581872, 584998
Fax: (62-24) 581872

PT Mustika Ratu
Gd. Graha Mustika Ratu. Lt. PH
Jalan Gatot Subroto KAV 74–75
Jakarta Selatan 12870
Indonesia
Tel: (62-21) 8306754/59
Fax: (62-21) 8306760
www.mustika-ratu.co.id
email: m_ratu@indo.net.id

PT Nyonya Meneer
Jalan Raden Patah 191–199
Semarang 50126

Central Java
Indonesia
Tel: (62-24) 547532, 551965
Fax: (62-24) 411375

Jakarta office
Tel: (62-21) 3901142
Fax: (62-21) 338107
www.nyonyameneer.com
email: ptnmjkt@nyonyameneer.co.id

PT Rumput Patimah
Jalan Jen. A. Yani Km 8,
8 Kertak Hanyar, Banjarmasin
South Kalimantan
Indonesia

PT Sari Enesis Indah
Jalan Rawa Sumur II
Blok DD No.16 Kawasan Industri
Pulogadung
Jakarta Timur
Indonesia
Tel: (62-21) 4609481/82/83

PT Sekar Ayu
Jalan Bumi Putra III/5 C
Cipinang Baru
Jakarta Timur
Indonesia

PT Sinde Budi Sentosa
Wisma SMR Lt 7
Jalan Yos Sudarso KAV. 89
Jakarta Utara
Indonesia
Tel: (62-21) 6507879
Fax: (62-21) 6508126

PT Tenaga Tani Farma
Jalan K.H. Sya'dan No.70
Kemanggisan-Palmerah
Jakarta Barat 11480
Indonesia
Tel: (62-21) 5480106, 5302748
Fax: (62-21) 5301473
email: tenagatani@dnet.net.id
www.tenagatani.com/index.html

OVERSEAS JAMU COMPANIES

AUSTRALIA
(Nyonya Meneer products)
c/o Mrs Gwyneth Roberts
46 Linckens Crescent
Balwyn
Victoria 3103
Australia
Tel (61-3) 98362966
Fax (61-3) 98362082

HONG KONG
(Martina Berto products)
c/o Fonson Limited
Room 3101–3102
31st Floor, Trendy Centre
682 Castle Peak Road
Cheung Wha Wan
Kowloon
Hong Kong

GERMANY
PT Nyonya Meneer
c/o Mr Peter Fries
Grenzwisch 9F
D-22359 Hamburg
Germany
Tel (49-40) 6045994
Fax (49-40) 6045600

KOREA
(Martina Berto products)
c/o Jamu Korea
7F Hanseng Building 1306–03
Seocho Dong
Seochoku
Seoul
Korea

THE NETHERLANDS
PT Jamu Indonesia Simona
Indo Art
Klaprozenweg 74, 1032 KX
Amsterdam
The Netherlands
Tel (31-20) 6341639

PT Nyonya Meneer
c/o Mr Satrijo
Nyonya Meneer Commercial Co
Dobal Straat 9
2718 Zoetermeer
The Netherlands
Tel (31-79) 617589

MALAYSIA
PT Jamu Indonesia Simona
Mulyana Sdn. Bhd
No. 11 & 15, Jalan TPP 1/15
Taman Industri Puchong
2, Jalan Puchong
47100 Selangor-Darul Ehsan
Malaysia
Tel (60-3) 571 5232

(Nyonya Meneer products)
c/o Mr Soepie Hj Ali Ipin,
Teras Perkasa Sdn. Bhd
No 19, Jalan 11A/133 Sri Sentosa
58000 Kuala Lumpur
Malaysia
Tel: (60-3) 794 1782
Fax: (60-3) 794 1793

Martina Berto (m) Sdn Bhd
No 65 Jalan Hujan
Overseas United Garden
58200 Kuala Lumpur
Malaysia

Wisma Mustika Ratu No. 18
Jalan 5/91A Taman Shamelin Perkasa
Batu 3 1/2 Jalan Cheras
56100 Kuala Lumpur
Malaysia
Tel: (60-3) 986 1626
Fax: (60-3) 983 6625

SINGAPORE
(Jamu Indonesia Simona and **Mustika Ratu)**
Fatimah Trading Enterprise
7 Jalan Pinang
Singapore 199139
Tel (65) 296 7083
Fax (65) 292 0744

SWITZERLAND
Jamu Borobudur
Berghofstrasse 18
CH-8421 Dattlikon
Switzerland
Tel/Fax (41-52) 315 1050

UNITED STATES
Collier & Collier Spas/
JAMU Asian Spa Rituals
6477 South 93rd Street
Whitefish
Montana 59937
USA
Tel (1-406) 862 2200, 863 2963
Fax (1-406) 863 2964
email: spacollier@aol.com (Cary Collier)
        kim@jamuspa.com (Kim Collier)
www.jamuspa.com

(Nyonya Meneer products)
c/o Mrs Wulan Naughton
Quest International
521 Ala Moana Blvd, STE 216
Honolulu
Hawaii 96813
Tel (1-808) 533 0331

PT Jamu Indonesia Simona
Premier Health Product
1320 Kalani Street, Suite 288
Honolulu
Hawaii
Tel (1-808) 848 4811

(Jamu Borobudur products)
Ms Sylvie S.
1806 Chantilly Lane
Fullerton
CA 92833
USA
Tel: (1-714) 2781770
www.asiareceipe.com

JAMU WEBSITES

www.joglosemar.co.id/jamu.html

www.geocities.com/tadrake/jamu.html

www.fao.org/decrep/xs336e/x5336e0u.htm

www.nuffic.nl/ciran/ikdm/
2-1/articles/sidik.html

www.puska.or.id/psbh/psbhair/abstrak1-10.htm

www.indoprogate.com/jamu/jamu.htm

www.margajaya.8m.com

www.indomerchant.com/medicine.html

www.balifolder.com/reference/trael/
13,05,02,02.shtml

www.Indonesianjamu.com

www.indonesia.elga.net.id

PLANT GLOSSARY

INDONESIAN	BOTANICAL	ENGLISH	PART USED
Akar tuba	Derris elliptica	Fish poison root	Root
Akar wangi	Vetiveria zizanioides	Vetiver	Root
American variety lengkuas	Alpinia officinarum	Lesser galangal	Rhizome
Asem	Tamarindus indica	Tamarind	Fruit pulp
Babakan pulai	Alstonia scholaris	Pulai tree	Bark
Bawang merah	Allium capa	Red onion	Bulb
Bawang putih	Allium sativum	Garlic	Bulb
Benalu	Loranthus sp.	Indian mistletoe	Leaf
Bengle	Zingiber cassumunar	Purple ginger	Rhizome
Beras	Oryza sativa	Raw white rice	Starch
Bidara laut (genuine)	Strychnos ignatii	White bitter wood	Wood
Bidara laut (Pasak bumi)	Eurycoma longifolia	Earth's peg	Root
Biji lamtoro	Leucaena glauca	Chinese petay tree	Seed
Botor	Pacphocarpus tetragonolobus	Four-sided bean	Seed
Buah salak	Salacca edulis	Snake fruit	Fruit
Bunga srigading	Nyctanthes arbor-tristis	Red white tree	Flower
Burahol	Stelechocarpus burahol	Fist tree	Fruit
Cabe besar	Capsicum annum	Green chilli	Fruit
Cabe jawa	Piper retrofractum	Javanese long pepper	Fruit
Cabe rawit	Capsicum frutescens	Small chilli	Fruit
Cendana	Santalum album	Sandalwood	Wood
Cempaka putih	Michelia sp.	Tropical white magnolia	Flower
Chengkeh	Syzgium aromatica	Clove	Bud
Cimera	Zingiber officinarum var. rubrum	Red ginger	Rhizome
Daoen inggoe	Ruta angustifolia	Silver leaf	Leaf
Daun bangkuwang	Pachyrrhizus erosus	Earth melon; yam bean	Leaf
Daun dewa	Gynura procumbens	Leaf of divinity	Leaf
Daun jengkol	Pithecellobium jiringa	Stinky bean	Leaf
Daun kates	Carica papaya	Papaya	Leaf
Daun miana	Coleus scutellarioides	Mayana	Leaf
Daun meniran/Dukung dukung anak	Phyllanthus niruri	Child pick-a-back	Leaf
Daun salam	Syzygium polyanthum	Kitchen bay	Leaf
Daun sendok	Plantago major	Cup leaves	Leaf
Daun sambiloto	Andrographis paniculata	Date leaf	Leaf
Duwet	Eugenia cumini	Java plum tree	Seed

Elung ubi jalar	Ipomoea batatas	Sweet potato	Young leaf
Gaharu	Aquilaria malaccensis	Aloewood	Wood
Gambir putih	Uncaria gambieri	White gambier	Leaf extract
Gandapura/Kasturi	Abelmoschus moschatus	Javanese musk mallow	Seed
Gandapura	Gaultheria procumbens	Wintergreen	Essential oil
Getah kasawe	Manihot utilissima	Cassava	Milky juice
Gula aren	Arenga pinnata	Palm sugar	Sugar
Gula batu	Saccharum officinarum	Rock sugar	Sugar
Gula jawa/Gula merah	Cocos nucifera	Coconut sugar	Sugar
Gurih	Hydrocotyle asiatica	Horse foot plant	Herb, leaf
Handeuleum	Graptophyllum pictum	Caricature plant	Leaf
Jahe	Zingiber officinale	Common ginger	Rhizome
Jahe merah	Zingiber officinale var. rubrum	Red ginger	Rhizome
Jambe	Areca catechu	Betel nut	Fruit
Jambu biji/ Jambu batu	Psidium guajava	Guava	Leaf
Jarak kosta	Jatropha curcas	Physic nut	Latex
Jati belanda	Guazuma ulmifolia	Bastard cedar tree	Leaf
Jenitri	Elaeocarpus ganitrus	Java laurel tree	Gall
Jeruk kingkit	Triphasia trifolia	Lime berry	Fruit
Jeruk nipis	Citrus aurantifolia	Thin skinned lime	Fruit
Jinten	Cuminum cyminum	Cumin	Seed
Jungrahab/ujung atap	Baeckea frutescens	Needle or roof edge tree	Leaf
Kacang mede	Anacardium occidentale	Cashew nut	Leaf, fruit
Kaki kuda	Centella asiatica	Indian pennywort	Leaf, herb
Kangkung	Ipomoea aquatica	Water convulvulus	Leaf
Kapulago	Elettaria cardamomum	Cardamon	Fruit
Kasawe/Ubi singkong	Manihot utilissima	Cassava	Starch
Kayu angin	Usnea thalus	Beard moss	Thallus
Kayu legi	Glycyrrhiza glabra	Chinese liquorice	Root
Kayu manis	Cinnamomum zeylanicum	Cinnamon	Bark
Kayu pahit	Strychnos ligustrina	Bitterwood tree	Wood
Kayu putih	Melaleuca leucadendra	Cajuput tree	Oil
Kayu rapet	Parameria laevigata	Stretch shrub	Bark
Kayu ular	Strychnos lucida	Snakewood	Wood
Kecambah kedelai hitam	Glycine max	Soybean (black variety)	Seed sprout
Kecubung	Datura metal	Horn of plenty	Leaf
Kecibeling	Sericocalyx crispus	Glass splinter leaf	Leaf
Kedawung	Parkia roxburghii	Giant Chinese petay tree	Seed

Kelembak	*Rheum sp.*	Java rhubarb	Root
Kembang pukul empat	*Mirabilis jalapa*	Four o'clock flower	Leaf
Kemiri	*Aleurites moluccana*	Candlenut	Seed
Kemukus	*Piper cubeba*	Cubeb pepper	Fruit
Kenanga	*Canangium odoratum*	Cananga, Ylang-ylang	Flower
Kencur	*Kaempferia galanga*	Resurrection lily	Rhizome
Kenikir	*Cosmos caudatus*	Yellow gardenia	Leaf
Kepel	*Stelechocarpus burahol*	Fist tree	Fruit
Ketumbar	*Coriandrum sativum*	Coriander	Leaf
Kikoneng	*Arcangelisia flava*	—	—
Kingkit	*Triphasia trifolia*	Lime berry	Fruit
Kluangan/Daun dilen	*Pogostemon cablin*	Patchouli	Leaf
Kulit pule	*Alstonia scholaris*	Pulai tree	Bark
Kumia kucing	*Orthosiphon aristatus*	Cat's whiskers	Leaf
Kunci pepet/Kunyit putih	*Kaempferia rotunda*	White turmeric	Rhizome
Kunir	*Curcuma domestica*	Long turmeric	Rhizome
Lada hitam	*Piper nigrum*	Black pepper	Fruit
Lada putih	*Piper nigrum*	White pepper	Seed
Lengkuas, laos	*Languas galanga*	Greater galangal	Rhizome
Legundi	*Vitex trifolia*	Indian privet	Leaf
Lempuyang pahit	*Zingiber amaricans*	Bitter ginger	Rhizome
Lempuyang wangi	*Zingiber aromaticum*	—	Rhizome
Lobak	*Raphanus sativus*	Giant white radish	Root
Luntas	*Pluchea indica*	Firefly shrub	Leaf
Manis jangan	*Cinnamomum burmanii*	Java cinnamon	Bark
Masoyi	*Cryptocarya massoy*	Massoi bark	Bark
Mata pelandok	*Ardisia elliptica*	Mouse deer's eye	Stem
Mengkudu	*Morinda citrifolia*	Indian mulberry	Leaf, fruit
Mungsi	*Artemisia absinthium*	Absinth or wormwood	Fruit
Nanas	*Ananas comosus*	Pineapple	Fruit
Orang-aring (Urang-aring)	*Eclipta prostrata*	False daisy	Leaf
Pala	*Myristica fragrans*	Nutmeg	Seed, mace
Pare	*Momordica charantia*	Bitter gourd, bitter melon	Leaf
Pasak bumi	*Eurycoma longifolia*	Earth's peg	Root
Patmosari	*Rafflesia patma*	Giant Rafflesia	Flower
Pinang	*Areca catechu*	Betelnut	Fruit
Pisang kepok	*Musa sp.*	Bird banana	Leaf, bulb

Pandan wangi	Pandanus amaryllifolius	Fragrant screwpine	Leaf
Pisang mas	Musa sp.	Gold banana	Leaf, bulb
Pisang raja	Musa sp.	King banana	Leaf, bulb
Pisang wangi	Musa sp.	Fragrant banana	Leaf, bulb
Pisang tanduk	Musa sp.	Horn plantain	Leaf, bulb
Pulai/Pule	Alstonia scholaris	Pulai tree	Bark
Pulosari	Alyxia stellata	Pulasari tree	Bark
Puoung	Pangium edule	Kluwak tree	Seed
Purwoceng	Pimpinella alpina	Man's power root	Root
Remujung	Orthosiphon aristatus	Cat's whiskers	Leaf
Sambiloto	Andrographis paniculata	Date leaf	Leaf
Sambung nyawa	Gynura procumbens	Life sustaining plant	Leaf
Semanggi/Calincing	Oxalis corniculata	Yellow club	Leaf
Sembukan	Paederia foetida	Stinky plant	Leaf
Seprantu	Sindora sumatrana	Prickly disk	Fruit
Sidowayah	Woodfordia fruticosa	Grandchild's arrival	Flower + leaf
Sintok	Cinnamomum sintoc	Sintoc tree	Bark
Sogo talik	Abrus precatorius	Bead plant	Leaf
Surti	Zingiber officinale var. rubrum	Small ginger	Rhizome
Sirih	Piper betle	Betel	Leaf
Tabat barito	Ficus deltoidea	Borneo fig tree	Leaf
Tapak dara	Catharanthus roseus	Madagaskar periwinkle	Leaf
Tapak liman	Elephantopus scaber	Elephant's foot	Leaf, root
Tempuyung	Sonchus arvensis		Leaf
Temu besar	Curcuma xanthorrhiza	Round turmeric	Rhizome
Temu ireng	Curcuma aeruginosa	Black turmeric	Rhizome
Temu giring	Curcuma heyneana	Shepherd turmeric	Rhizome
Temu kunci	Boesenbergia pandurata	Key turmeric	Rhizome
	Gastrochilus panduratum		
Temu kuning	Curcuma zedoaria	Long or round zedoary	Rhizome
Temu mangga	Curcuma mangga	Mango turmeric	Rhizome
Temu lawak	Curcuma xanthorrhiza	Round turmeric	Rhizome
Temu putih	Kaempferia rotunda	White turmeric	Rhizome
Urip	Euphorbia tirucalli	Milk bush of Finger tree	Bark, leaf
Widuri	Calotropis gigantea	Mudar plant	Bark, leaf

BIBLIOGRAPHY

A

Abdulkadir B.
Buku Masakan & Jamu Tradisional, Yogyakarta, 1992

Alexander, Jane
Supertherapies, Bantam Books, Great Britain, 1996

Anselmo, Peter with James S. Brooks, M.D.
Ayurvedic Secrets to Longevity & Total Health, Prentice Hall, New Jersey

Airlangga University
IASTAM Proceedings—the Second International Congress on Traditional Asian Medicine, Airlangga University Surabaya, Indonesia, September 2–7, 1984

Asmino
Pengalaman Pribadi Dengan Pengobatan Alternatif, Kongres Nasional II, Perhimpunan Onkologi Indonesia (POI), Surabaya, 1993

B

Back, Philippa
The Illustrated Herbal: The Complete Guide to Growing and Using Herbs, Chancellor Press, London, 1996

Barbier, Christine, Courvoisier, Christian
An Approach of the Traditional Uses of Medicinal Plants in Java, Diplome D'Etudes Approfondies D'Ecologie Generale et Appliquee, Academie de Montpellier, 1980

Beekman E.M.
The Poison Tree. Selected Writings of Rumphius on the Natural History of the Indies, Edited and Translated by E.M. Beekman, Oxford University Press, Kuala Lumpur, 1993

Bevan Dr James
A Pictorial Handbook of Anatomy and Physiology, Universal International, Gordon, NSW, Australia, 1997

Bremness, Lesley
The Complete Book of Herbs: A Practical Guide to Growing & Using Herbs, Viking Studio Books, Penguin Books USA Inc, 1994

Brierley, Joanna Hall
Spices, The Story of Indonesia's Spice Trade, Oxford University Press, Kuala Lumpur, 1994

Bown, Deni
The Royal Horticultural Society Encyclopedia of Herbs and their Uses, Dorling Kindersley, London 1995

Bradford, Nikki (Consultant Editor)
The Hamlyn Encyclopedia of Complementary Health, Hamlyn, London, 1996

Burkill, I.H.
A Dictionary of the Economic Products of the Malay Peninsula Vol. I & II, Kuala Lumpur, Malaysia, Ministry of Agriculture and Co-operatives, 1966

Burbidge F.W.
The Gardens of the Sun—A Naturalist's Journal of Borneo & the Sulu Archipelagi, Singapore, Oxford University Press, 1991

C

Caddick, Helen
Plants in the Arts and Culture of Indonesia, paper presented to Ganeshe Study Group, 1989

Carper, Jean
The Food Pharmacy Guide to Good Eating, Bantam Books, USA, 1991

Chevallier, Andrew
The Encyclopedia of Medicinal Plants, London, Dorling Kindersley, 1996

Clevely Andi, Richmond Katherine
The Complete Book of Herbs, Read Publications Incorporated, Toronto, Canada, 1995

D

Darmi, Soeparto
Jamu in the Health & Beauty of the Javanese Woman

Departmen Kesehatan RI
Tanaman Obat Indonesia Jilid I & II, Jakarta, Departmen Kesehatan Republik Indonesia, 1985

Departmen Kesehatan RI
Permanfaatan Tanaman Obat, Edisi II, Departmen Kesehatan Republik Indonesia, 1989

Dr. Dharma, A.P
Indonesian Medical Plants, Jakarta, Balai Pustaka, 1987

E

Eisai
Medicinal Herb Index in Indonesia, P.T. Eisai, Indonesia, 1986

Eiseman, Fred and Margaret
Fruits of Bali, Periplus Editions, Singapore, 1994

F

Farr, Maria/Wood, Marilyn
Jamu Tour, Heritage Society Library, Jakarta, 1991

Florida, Nancy. K.
Javanese Literature in Surakarta Manuscripts Vol. I, Itaca: Cornell University Southeast Asia Programme, 1993

H

Hall, Dorothy
Herbal Medicine, Thomas C Lothian Pty Ltd, PortMelbourne, Australia, 1994

Hall, Julia Clare
Managing the Rainforest, Swiddens, Housegardens and Trade in Central Kalimantan, Project Baritu Ulu, 1993

Hargono, Djoko
Pemanfaatan Tanaman Obat untuk Kesehatan Keluarga, Departmen Pendidikan dan Kebudayaan dengan PT Rineka, Cipta, Januari 1993

Harsrinuksmo, Bambang
Pijat dan Urut Cara Jawa, Jakarta, Grafikatama Jaya, 1992

Hembing Wijayakusuma, H.M
Tanaman Berkhasiat Obat di Indonesia Jilid Ke 1–4, Pustaka Kartini, Jakarta, 1992–1995

Heinerman, John
Heinerman's Encyclopedia of Fruits, Vegetables and Herbs, Reward Books, Parker Publishing Company, West Nyack, New York, USA, 1988

Hose Charles
Natural Man—Record from Borneo, Singapore, Oxford University Press, 1990

Hose, Charles
The Fieldbook of a Jungle Wallah, Oxford University Press, Asia, 1985

Hutton, Wendy
Tropical Herbs & Spices of Malaysia & Singapore, Periplus Editions, Singapore, 1997

I

Idrus H.A.
Terapi Pijat & Urut: spesialis untuk kebugaran, kecantikan, peremajaan dan kejantanan, CV Aneka, Solo, 1995

Indonesian Parenthood Association
Report on the Study of Dukuns in Central Java, 1971

J

Jordaan, Roy. E
Folk Medicine in Madura (Indonesia), Madura Research Project, Dutch-Indonesian Project for the Promotion of Indonesian Studies, Leiden, 1985

K

Karkono Kamajaya. H
Serat Centhini—Relavansinya dengan Masa Kini, Jakarta, Balai Pustaka, 1988

Kloppenburg-Versteegh. J
Wenken en Raadgevingen Betreffende het Gebruik van Indische Planten Vruchten, Enz. Semarang Servire Katwijk, 1934

L

LeShan, Laurence
How To Meditate, Thorsons, London, 1995

Lucas, Richard, M.
Miracle Medicine Herbs, Parker Publishing Company, West Nyack, New York, USA, 1991

Lucas, Richard
Secrets of the Chinese Herbalists, Parker Publishing Company, West Nyack, New York, USA, 1977

Lumholtz, Carl
Through Central Borneo, Oxford in Asia Paperbacks

M

Mann, Richard & Jenny
Helping the Indonesian Dream Come True: Women's Role in Development, Gateway Books, Toronto, Ortario, Canada, 1994

Mann, Richard I
Marine Tourism: Indonesia, Gateway Books, Toronto, Ontario, Canada, 1994

Mardisiswojo, Sudarman/Rajakmangunsudarso, Harsono
Cabe Puyang Warisan Nenek Moyang, PN Balai Pustaka, Jakarta, 1985

Marhijanto, Bambang
Methode Penyembuhan Alami Melalui Pijat Refleksi 2, Bintang Timur, Surabaya

McIntyre, Anne
Herbs for Common Ailments, Gaia Books Limited, London, 1992

Mindell, Earl
The Herb Bible, Vermilion, London, 1994

Ministry of Health, Republic of Indonesia
Utilization of Medicinal Plants, Ministry of Health Republic of Indonesia, 1981

N

Norman, Jill
The Complete Book of Spices—A Practical Guide to Spices and Aromatic Seeds, Dorling Kindersley, London, 1991

O

Ody, Penelope
The Herb Society's Complete Medicinal Herbal, Dorling Kindersley, London, 1993

Olsen, Kirsten
Alternative Health Care: The Encyclopedia of Choices in Healing, Chancellor Press, London, 1994

Owen, Sri
Indonesian Regional Food & Cookery, Doubleday, London, 1994

P

Paton, Vicki Anne
Thesis; Healing in a Central Javanese Village, University of Western Australia, 1988

Periplus World Cookbooks
The Food of Indonesia: Authentic Recipes from the Spice Islands, Periplus Editions, Singapore, 1995

Periplus World Cookbooks
The Food of Bali: Authentic Recipes from the Island of the Gods, Periplus Editions, Singapore, 1995

Periplus Adventure Guides
Bali: Indonesia, Periplus Editions (HK) Ltd, 1995

Perry , Lily M.
Medicinal Plants of East and Southeast Asia: Attributed Properties and Uses, The MIT Press, Cambridge, Massachusetts, USA, 1980

Pigeaud, Theodore G.Th.
Literature of Java: Catalogue Raisonne of Javanese Manuscripts in the Library of the University of Leiden & Other Public Collections in the Netherlands. Nijhoff & Leiden University Press 1967–1980

Piper, Jacqueline M.
Fruits of South-East Asia: Facts and Folklore, Oxford University Press, Singapore, 1989

Polunin, Mirian & Robbins, Christopher
The Natural Pharmacy: An Encyclopedic Illustrated Guide to Medicines from Nature, Dorling Kindersley, London, 1992

Ponder, H.W.
Javanese Panorama, More Impressions of the 1930's, Oxford University Press, Singapore, 1990

R

Rahman, Fazlur
Health and Medicine in the Islamic Tradition, Malaysia, S Abdul Majeed & Co, 1993

Reader's Digest
Magic and Medicine of Plants, The Reader's Digest Association, Inc, New York/Montreal, 1993

Riswan, S. & Sangat-Roemantyo, Harini
Javanese Traditional Cosmetics from Plants, Medicinal Products from Tropical Rainforests, Forest Research Institute of Malaysia May 13–15, Kuala Lumpur, Malayia 1991

Riswan.S and Sangat-Roemantyo. H
Ethnobotanical and Social Aspects of Traditional Medicine, Bioresources— Diversity, Ethnobiology, Development and Sustainability, International Centenary Conference, University of Western Sydney July 15–17, 1991

Rooneu, Dawn F.
Betel Chewing Traditions in South-East Asia, Oxford University Press, Kuala Lumpur, 1993

Rumphius
The Poison Tree, translated by EM Beekman, OAP, 1993

S

Sangat-Roemantyo, Harini & Soeparto, Soedarmilah
Jamu in the Past, at Present and in the Future, IInd ICTAM Conference in Surabaya, Indonesia 2–7 September 1984

Sangat-Roemantyo, Harini
Short Notes on Jamu, Jamu Gendong and Jamu Factories

Sangat-Roemantyo, Harini & S. Riswan
Utilization of Wild Medicinal Plants and its Conservation: A Case Study in Java, The Asean Workshop on Wildlife Research and Management and The Meeting on Establishment of Asean Wildlife Society, Bogor, Directorate General of Forest Protection and Nature Conservation, Ministry of Forestry, 1990

Sangat-Roemantyo, Harini
Ethnobotany of the Javanese Incense, Economic Botany, The Society for Economic Botany by The New York Botanical Gardens, Issue 4, September 1990

Sangat-Roemantyo, Harini & Soedarsono Riswan
Javanese Medicinal Plants: Their Distribution and Uses, International Congress on Traditional Medicines and Medicinal Plants, Denpasar, Bali, October 15–17, 1990

Santa, IGP
Medicinal Plants of Bali & Java, International Congress on Traditional Medicine and Medicinal Plants, October 15–17, Denpasar, Bali, Indonesia, Laboratory of Pharmaceutical Botany, Pharmacognosy, Faculty of Pharmacy, Airlangga University, Surabaya, 1990

Santoso, Prof. Dr. Sardjono Oerip
Perkembangan Obat Tradisional Dalam Ilmu Kedokteran di Indonesia dan Upaya Pengebangannya Sebagai Obat Alternatif, Jakarta, 1993

Schauenberg, Paul/Paris, Ferdinand
Guide to Medicinal Plants, Guildford and London, Lutterworth Press, 1977

Author/s Unknown
Serat Centhini (Suluk Tambangraras) Jilid 1–12; Yogyakarta, Yayasan Centhini, 1992

Shealy, Norman C (Consultant Editor)
The Complete Family Guide to Alternative Medicine: An Illustrated Encyclopedia of Natural Healing, Element Books, Shaftesbury, Dorset, 1996

Stockwell, Christine
Nature's Pharmacy: A History of Plants and Healing, Published in association with the Royal Botanic Gardens, Kew and Century, London, undated

Stuart, Malcolm
The Encyclopedia of Herbs and Herbalism, edited by Malcolm Stuart, Black Cat for Bookmart Limited, Leicester, UK, 1994

Suprana, Jaya
A Short Introduction to Jamu, the Indonesian Traditional Way to Beauty, Health & Happiness, Cap Jago

Suparto, Darmi
JAMU in the Health & Beauty Care of the Javanese Woman, Jamu Darmi, November 1974

Sutarjadi, Prof.
Traditional Medicine in Indonesia. Differences and Similarities in Basic Concepts compared with Chinese Traditional Medicine, Surabaya, Faculty of Pharmacy Airlangga University, 1991. Paper; 2nd World Congress of Chinese Medicine & Pharmacy, Taipei, 1986

Sutarjadi, Prof.
Masalah Obat Asli Indonesia. Faculty of Pharmacy Air Langga University, Paper; Ceramah Ilmiah pada Kongres National isfi de Jakarta, 1967

Sutrisno, Drs. R. Bambang
Pengembangan Fitofarmaka di Indonesia, Paper Seminar Indonesian RRC Traditional Medicine Expos '93 di Gedung Asemka, Jakarta, 1993

Dra Syamsuhidayat/Sri Sugati/Hutapea, Dr. Johnny Ria
Inventaris Tanaman Obat Indonesia (I), (II), (III), Jakarta Departmen Kesehatan RI, Badan Penelitian dan Pengembangan Kesehatan 1991–1994

Dra Segatri, Putra
Taru Premana. Bali, Upada Sastra, 1989

Suryani, Luh Ketut/Jensen, Gordon D.
Trance and Possession in Bali: A Window on Western Multiple Personality, Possession Disorder, and Suicide, Oxford University Press, Kuala Lumpur, Malaysia. 1993

T

Tilaar, M, Sangat-Roemantyo H & S Riswan
Kunyit (Curcuma Domestica) The Queen of Jamu Products from Tropical Rainforests, Forest Research Institute of Malaysia May 13–15, Kuala Lumpur, Malayia 1991

Tamin, Yusuf, M.
Dari Cultuurtuin Hingga Pusat Penelitian dan Pengembangan Tanaman Industri Bogor 1876–1988, Balai Penelitian Tanaman Rempah dan Obat, Bogor, 1988

Trattler, Ross
Better Health Through Natural Healing, Thorsons, London, 1987

U

Author/s unknown
Usada Tua (Terjemahan) Ciri Lontar: No.III.d.956/10
Bali, Gedong Kirtya Singaraja

V

Van Beek, Aart
Life in the Javanese Kraton, Oxford University Press, Singapore, 1990

Veevers-Carter, W.
Riches of the Rainforest, Oxford University Press, Singapore, 1991

W

Wall, Kaarin
A Jakarta Market, American Women's Association, Jakarta, Indonesia, 1985

Walujojati, Harsasi
Pijat Tradisional, Bintang Usaha Jaya, Surabaya

Prof. Wee Yeow Chin
A Guide to Medicinal Plants, Omni Theatre, Singapore Science Centre, Singapore, 1992

WHO
Medicinal Plants in China, World Health Organisation, Regional Office for Western Pacific, Manila, 1989

Y

Yen Ho, Alice
At the South-East Asian Table, Oxford University Press, Kuala Lumpur, 1995